healing
MIND
healing
BODY

healing
MIND
healing
BODY

explaining how the mind and body work together

debbie shapiro

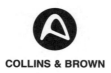

COLLINS & BROWN

Copyright ©Vega 2002
Text copyright © Debbie Shapiro 2002

First published in 2002 by Vega
This issue published in 2007 by
Collins & Brown
151 Freston Road
London
W10 6TH

An imprint of Anova Books Company Ltd

Distributed in the United States and Canada by
Sterling Publishing Co, 387 Park Avenue South, New York, NY 10016, USA

ISBN: 9 78184 340 407 1

A CIP catalogue record for this book is available from the British Library.

10 9 8 7 6 5 4 3 2 1

Printed and bound by Creative Print and Design, Ebbw Vale, Wales

This book can be ordered direct from the publisher.
Contact the marketing department, but try your bookshop first.

www.anovabooks.com

I dedicate this book to all my teachers
both past and present, including
my husband, Eddie Brahmananda Shapiro.
Thank you.

Contents

CHAPTER 1

The Body of Great Wisdom

Every exaggeration has its effect in the human body.

WALT WHITMAN

IN all the wonderful work being done in the field of medicine and healing, there is one basic concept that is often dismissed as irrelevant. That is the relationship between the mind and the body, and the possibility that this relationship might have a direct effect on either our state of health or our ability to heal. That this relationship does exist, and is actually of great importance, is only slowly coming to light; a true understanding of its deeper implications has yet to emerge and gain acceptance. Yet as we explore the extraordinary interplay of energies between the many aspects of our personality – our needs, unconscious reactions, repressed emotions, aspirations and fears – with the functioning of our physical system and its capacity to maintain itself, we soon realise how very wise the body is. With its intricately detailed systems and operations it portrays infinite intelligence and compassion, constantly giving us the means to understand ourselves further, to confront issues we are not looking at, and to go beyond that which is holding us back. For as much as our bodies manifest our conscious thoughts and feelings, so too they manifest the unconscious energies which underlie our every action.

To understand this bodymind connection, we first have to recognise that the mind and body are one. Generally we regard the body as something we carry about with us (often somewhat reluctantly), something that is easily damaged, that needs exercise, regular food and water, a certain amount of sleep and occasional check-ups. The body becomes a great nuisance when it is damaged, so then we take it to a doctor in the belief that he or she will be able to mend it, and the quicker the better. Something is broken, so we go to get it fixed – as if this 'something' is an inanimate object, devoid of intelligence. When the body is functioning well we are happy, we feel alive and energetic. When it is not, we soon become irritated, frustrated, depressed and full of self-pity.

This view of the body is sadly limited. It denies the complexity of the energies that make up our entire being, energies that are constantly communicating and flowing between each other; between our thoughts, feelings, and the physical maintenance of our various parts. There is no separation between what is happening in our minds and what is happening in our bodies; relatively we do not exist separate to the body in which we have our existence. Consider how in the English language we think of someone with great presence as a 'somebody', while a person with little significance is a 'nobody'. Our bodies are us; our state of being is a direct result of the communication between the numerous different aspects of our existence. To say 'I have hurt my arm', is to say that 'a hurt inside me is manifesting in my arm'. What the hurt in the arm is expressing is not different from verbal expressions of anger or confusion. To say there is a difference is to ignore the essential unity of the whole being. To treat only the arm is to disregard the source of the pain that the arm is manifesting. Denying this bodymind relationship is ignoring the opportunity that the body gives us to look at, accept and resolve our inner pain.

The effect of the bodymind relationship is easy to demonstrate. We know how feeling anxious or nervous about something can give rise to an upset stomach, constipation or a headache, or we become more accident-prone. We know that stress can lead to ulcers or even heart attacks; that depression and unhappiness make our bodies feel heavy and lethargic – we have little energy, we lose our appetite or eat excessively, get backache or tense shoulders. Meanwhile joyfulness and happiness increase our vitality and energy: needing less sleep and feeling more alive, we are also less likely to catch a cold or other infection as our bodies are stronger and therefore have greater resistance. However, we can take this bodymind understanding a great deal further to see how it can encompass all aspects of our physical and psychological life. We begin to understand that what happens to us physically is something over which we do have control, that we are not just a victim of, or have to suffer until it passes. What we experience within our bodies is an integral part of our whole being.

This concept of the bodymind is based on the belief in the unity and integrity of each human being: that though there are many different aspects that make up a whole person, these aspects cannot be isolated from each other, but are in constant relationship with, and have intimate knowledge of, each other at all times. The bodymind matrix reflects psychological and somatic harmony: the body is simply a gross manifestation of the subtlety of the mind. 'The skin is not separate from the emotions, or the emotions separate from the back, or the back separate from the kidneys, or the kidneys separate from will and ambition, or will and ambition separate from the spleen, or the spleen separate from sexual confidence,' wrote Dianne Connelly in *Traditional Acupuncture: The Law of the Five Elements*.

This complete unity of body and mind is reflected in our state of wellness and illness. Each state is a means which the bodymind has of giving us an indication of what is going on beneath the surface. For instance, illnesses or accidents often come at times of great change, such as moving home, a new marriage, or getting a different job. The inner conflicts at such times of change easily upset our balance and give rise to uncertainty and fear. This leaves us open and vulnerable to invading bacteria or viruses. At the same time, becoming ill then gives us a period of rest, time to realign and adjust to the changes. An illness is telling us that we need to stop doing something: it gives us the space in which to connect with those parts of us with which we are out of touch. It also puts things in perspective, such as the importance of our relationships and communication. In this way we can see the wisdom of the bodymind in action, the mind and body constantly affecting and working with each other.

Conveying the messages from our minds to our bodies is an intricate system comprised of the bloodstream, the nervous system, and numerous hormones secreted by the endocrine glands. It is an extraordinarily complex process, regulated by the pituitary gland and the hypothalamus. The hypothalamus is a small region in the brain that maintains many of the body's functions such as temperature and heartbeat, as well as the sympathetic and para-sympathetic nerve functioning. Numerous nerve fibres from all over the brain are linked to the hypothalamus, and in this way it connects psychological and emotional activity with bodily functioning. For instance, the vegas nerve from the hypothalamus connects directly to the stomach – hence stomach problems in relation to stress or anxiety; while other nerves connect to the thymus and the spleen, which in turn make the immune cells and regulate the immune functioning in the blood.

The immune system is extremely powerful in its ability to protect by rejecting that which is harmful to us, but it is also subject to brain dominance via the nervous system. It is therefore directly affected by psychological stress. When we suffer severe stress of any kind, then the hormones released by the adrenal glands will disrupt the brain-immune system relationship and actually suppress the immune system, leaving us vulnerable to illness and disease. Stress is not the only factor that can trigger this response. Negative reactions, such as repressed or prolonged anger, hatred, bitterness or depression, as well as loneliness or intense grieving, can also suppress the immune system by stimulating an over-production of these hormones.

In the brain we also find the limbic system, a grouping of structures which includes the hypothalamus. It has two major functions: to regulate autonomic functioning such as fluid balance, gastro-intestinal activity and endocrine secretion, and also to integrate the emotions: it has even been called the 'seat of the emotions' in man. Limbic activity links our emotional state and balance with the endocrine and hormone system, so it is obviously a major player in the bodymind relationship. Input for limbic activity and hypothalamus functioning appears to come directly from the cerebral cortex; this part of the brain is responsible for all our intellectual activity, including thinking, memory, perception and interpretation.

It is from the cerebral cortex that the alarm will be sounded whenever there is any form of perceived life-threatening activity. (Perceived is not always the same as actual life-threatening. For instance, stress is perceived by the body as life-threatening, even though we may think it is not.) The alarm signal then affects the limbic and hypothalamus organisation, which in turn affect the hormone secretion, and the immune and nervous systems. As these become alerted to danger, it is little wonder that the rest of the body is also affected, leading to tense muscles, nervous disarray, constricted blood vessels, and organ and cellular malfunction.

Before we too become alarmed by reading this, we need to

remember that it is not the event itself that is causing this response, but our reaction to the event. As Shakespeare said: There is nothing either good or bad, but thinking makes it so.' Stress is our psychological reaction to an event; it is not the event itself. And it is not a quick and soon forgotten flash of anger or despair that will set off the alarm system – it is the cumulative effect of constant or long-repressed negative emotion that will do it. The longer the unacknowledged state of mind is maintained, the more damage it can do as it wears down the bodymind resistance and constantly gives out a negative life message.

However, there is always room for change, as we can always work with ourselves and go from reacting to responding, from being subjective to being objective. For instance, if we live or work in a place where we are constantly subject to a great deal of noise, we can react by becoming increasingly irritated, getting tense headaches and high blood pressure; or we can respond objectively to the situation and look for positive solutions. The message we give our bodies – one of irritation or acceptance – is the message to which our bodies will answer. The repetition of negative thought patterns and attitudes such as worry, guilt, jealousy, anger, criticism, fear, and so on are likely to cause us far more harm than any external situation can. Our entire nervous system is under the control of a 'central regulatory agency', the control centre that in man we call the personality. In other words, the situations in our lives are neither negative nor positive – they just are. It is our personal reaction or response to them that labels them as one thing or another.

Our bodies reflect the events and experiences we have had in the way they move, function and operate; we are the sum total of all that has happened to us. The body actually retains everything it has ever experienced – all the events, emotions, stresses and pains are locked within the bodily system. A good bodymind therapist can read a person's entire life history by looking at the formation and shape of the body, its ability to move freely or with constriction, areas of tension, as well as the types of accidents, illnesses or diseases that have happened. Our bodies become like a walking autobiography, muscle and flesh formations reflecting our experiences, injuries, worries, anxieties and attitudes. Whether we have a timid posture – one that is bowed over and depressed or one that is standing square and defensive, all are learnt and adapted to early in life and become

built into our very structure. To believe that the body is a
separately operating, purely mechanical organism is to miss the
point entirely. It is to deny ourselves this source of great wisdom
that is available at all times.

In the same way that the body reflects what is happening in the
mind, so the mind is then subject to the pain and discomfort
being expressed in the body. There can be no escaping the
universal law of karma, that of cause and effect. For every effect
in our lives, there has to have been a cause. For every effect in our
bodies, there is a thought pattern or emotional state that
preceded it. In the words of Paramahansa Yogananda,

> There is an innate connection between the mind and the body.
> Whatever you hold in your mind will be produced in the physical
> body. Any ill-feeling or bitterness towards another person, intense
> passion, long-standing envy, corroding anxiety, fits of hot temper, all
> actually destroy the cells of the body and induce diseases of the heart,
> liver, kidneys, spleen, stomach, etc. Worry and stress have caused
> new deadly illnesses, such as high blood pressure, heart troubles,
> nervous breakdowns and cancer. All diseases have their origins in
> the mind. The pains that affect the physical body are secondary
> diseases.

To isolate the effect (the state of illness in the body) as being
unconnected to anything else is to deny the cause. In that case,
the cause (the underlying feelings and attitudes) will make
another effect known at some other time: another area of disease
or discomfort will arise in an attempt to show us where we are
out of balance.

The messages we unconsciously give our bodies are thus a
determining factor in our state of wellness. Messages based on
failure, despair and anxiety are ones that present a negative,
dying feeling and will cause the body to react by breaking down
the defence mechanisms (that is, the immune system) and
preparing for death. Even if our worries and fears are imaginary,
the message will still translate into physical illness as our bodies
feel endangered and threatened. To quote Shakespeare again,
'Cheerfulness is health; the opposite, melancholy, is disease.' If
we talk about our heart as being broken, does the body know the
difference between an emotionally broken heart and a physically
broken one? It appears not, as the power of the image in our mind
immediately affects the physical being. Research has repeatedly

shown how people often die shortly after the loss of a loved one, that they are basically dying of a broken heart. 'Can anxiety lead to serious illness?' asked Lawrence LeShan in *You Can Fight for Your Life*. 'Many medical investigators contend that there is hardly a major illness that cannot be triggered by profound anxiety. Depression and despair make their registrations not just in the mind but in the body.' We are expressing these more hidden and denied messages all the time, usually without being aware of them, for the unconscious is far more powerful in expressing our true feelings than is our conscious mind. These unconscious energies permeate all aspects of our lives.

Our everyday language describes this beautifully. To say that someone is 'a pain in the neck' can soon become a reality with stiff shoulders, neckache or headache; ambivalence becomes a 'splitting headache'; while 'a pain in the arse' can result in constipation or bowel cancer. Just as 'you've broken my heart' can lead to great despair, depression or coronary disease and is a dying message to the body, so 'this problem is eating me up alive' will often lead to stomach ulcers or intestinal difficulties. The more the body receives dying messages, the less it will be able to rally its defences and the means to survive.

When we acknowledge what is happening and take the time to look within, the body hears that we really do want to live; consequently it can respond and is able to start healing the inner pains and stresses. Messages based on joy, success, hope, love and wellness are living messages that encourage the body to build up its strength and vitality, to enter into full living.

However, on a conscious level we often pretend to both ourselves and others that all is fine – no worries, everything is just as it should be, there is nothing wrong at all. Few of us are willing to admit that we are frightened or lonely, feel tremendous guilt, or are angry and bitter. These are socially unacceptable qualities and therefore carefully repressed: 'Denial can follow us into the grave. Not only does the mind have strategies for walling off psychological conflict; it can also deny the illnesses that result from the first round of denial', wrote Marilyn Ferguson in *The Aquarian Conspiracy*. Our denied and repressed fears, worries and insecurities can all be found in the unconscious. It is from here that the body receives its messages, for it is the unconscious, and therefore the repressed attitudes and patterns, that affect our wellbeing.

Until the nineteenth century, the state of mind of a patient was of great importance to doctors; the psychosomatic connection between despair, depression, anger or grief, and debilitating illnesses was a clear one. As Dr Bernie Siegal says in *Love, Medicine and Miracles*, 'Contentment used to be considered a prerequisite for health.' Yet how many doctors nowadays will ask us if we are content and happy with our lives when we go to them with a backache or a kidney infection? And they would think us as a little mad if we were to start asking them about this bodymind relationship. The term psychosomatic has acquired a negative connotation, as it is invariably used to mean 'imaginary'. When doctors are unable to find a physical cause for a problem, and in order to release themselves from their responsibilities they conveniently label that problem as being 'all in the mind', purely imaginary, faked, or else the patient must be crazy. This attitude is due solely to the ignorance of the role that the mind plays in creating our reality.

The same misconceptions surround the idea of a placebo effect which is when a dummy medication (such as sugar water) is used, and yet the patient still gets well. Most doctors use the placebo as a trick to prove themselves right with people who they think are faking or imagining their illnesses. Paradoxically, if we see how all malfunctions in the body are a result of the mind, then there is no such thing as an isolated physical problem. The true meaning of the word psychosomatic – that the mind can influence the body – therefore applies to all physical states. As Dr Franz Alexander, a Chicago doctor, said some thirty years ago, 'Theoretically every disease is psychosomatic, since emotional factors influence all body processes through nervous and humoral pathways'. The placebo simply stimulates an activity that was in the mind all along – the desire to be well; the brain then releases a natural analgesic in response to our belief in our intrinsic wellness.

The only branch of conventional medicine that is really involved in understanding how the mind works in keeping us healthy or ill is PNI: psychoneuroimmunology. This grand name was developed after recognising the role of the mind (psycho) and the immune system (immunology), in relation to the nervous system (neuro). Nowadays, more and more varied professionals are exploring PNI, so at long last what is obvious to the irrational mind, the rational mind is beginning to prove! Unfortunately, however, the medical world in general is not interested in exploring or acknowledging the bodymind relationship. And the use of powerful drugs that has escalated so enormously in the last few decades has further robbed patients of their own healing authority.

Albert Schweitzer said, 'Each patient carries his own doctor inside him. We are best when we give the doctor who resides within each patient a chance to go to work.' But gone are the days when we used to heal ourselves at home with hot herbal teas and plenty of rest. We have become powerless and dependent, losing contact with our inner voice of intuition. Time in a doctor's surgery has been reduced to a quick check of symptoms and the writing of a prescription. It is not surprising therefore that we frequently return to our doctor with recurring symptoms, or even with new problems. How can there be real healing in these circumstances, when so little time is given to a visit and when the cause of the problem, the inner state of the patient, is being ignored? As doctors rarely have the time or the inclination to delve into our personal states, then obviously we are the ones who should be doing it.

Our physical malfunctions, on whatever level – whether they be from an accident, infection or stress – are the messages we can heed. When we become ill or develop a physical difficulty, we should first check the six to nine months leading up to the onset of the symptoms. Invariably we will find a clue during this time period. What emotional state was being experienced? Was there a big change in lifestyle? Excess stress or worry? A shift in circumstances, or unexpected misfortune? An accumulation of anger or frustration? From the recent past we can begin to look back further, to events from the distant past that we may still be carrying with us. The event itself may have gone, but the emotional impact can stay with us for many years and become ingrained in our bodies, finally affecting us on the cellular level.

It is not always easy to find the deeper cause of our patterns and attitudes, for they are often very carefully locked up. Looking at our childhood is one of the keys to understanding what is happening now. Were there any particular difficulties or strong feelings? Times of death, separation or similar trauma can leave deep imprints of fear, loss, grief, anger and insecurity. These stay with us, influencing and underlying our actions, behaviour, feelings and states of mind. It is staggering to see how many of us came from unhappy or unloved childhoods. Maybe our parents wanted a boy instead of a girl, or we were a mistake; perhaps we grew up listening to arguments and fighting; or we were caught in a divorce and spent our early years going back and forth between two parents who were hardly speaking to each other. These experiences undermine our sense of security, worthiness and acceptance. Childhood fears soon become adult fears. In time these begin to affect our health.

However, discovering the hidden emotional states that have caused our present predicaments does not mean to say that we can simply shrug our shoulders and blame our present state on something that happened in the past. The reason we are sick now is because those events, decisions or experiences are still with us. Seven million red blood cells die and are reformed every second. Every seven years our bones are fully rebuilt. Yet why are our cells re-formed in the same pattern as before if that pattern is not a healthy one? Is it because the inner programming has not changed? Because the mental behaviour patterns that are underlying our physical difficulties have not been affected? Is it because there are hidden, unexpressed reasons as to why we are ill, reasons that create a pay-off? To work with our inner programming in order to bring about change means going deep within to where our well-rooted convictions, prejudices, neuroses and idiosyncrasies lie. It is a serious business and not something that everyone will feel prepared to do.

Pain, illness or the malfunction of our bodies can therefore be seen as a message that we have a conflict of emotions and thoughts that is threatening our survival. This is not God's way of punishing us for all the terrible things we have done; it is our own way of creating balance out of imbalance. As we develop our understanding of the bodymind relationship, so we can ask, 'Why am I hurting myself in this way?' Consciously we do not want to beat ourselves up or experience pain and illness, yet that is what appears to be happening. When we recognise that the body is expressing what lies beneath the surface, that it is a mirror for us to look in to see our inner selves, and at the same time we truly recognise how all life is constantly aiming at fulfilment and balance, then we can see how our illnesses are our means to find that balance. Our difficulties are the maps and guides to finding the deeper levels of wisdom and unconditional love that are inherent within us all.

So rather than become overwhelmed by a sense of hopelessness and guilt that we are responsible for everything that is happening, we can see our illnesses as a tremendous challenge and opportunity for growth. Imbalance is a warning signal from our minds, a red alert for attention, the creation of an opportunity for us to learn and grow. Instead of feeling sorry or blaming ourselves, we can be more constructive, recognising our participation in both our illness and therefore also our wellness. Then we can ask, 'What is it that is needed here to enable my difficulties to be free to go?'

Thought that is intentional in its purpose directs energy, therefore energy follows thought. Wherever the thought is focused, there the energy will become concentrated. If we are considering our illness, and our thoughts and sensations are ones of being overwhelmed, then the illness may soon overwhelm us. If the energy thus becomes obstructed through the nature of the thought, then the blocked energy flow begins to cause discomfort, pain or disease. The energy flow is freed by a shift in our attitude to one of acceptance and freedom from stressful reaction, so the pain and discomfort can be eased. As Gaston St Pierre and I wrote in *The Metamorphic Technique*,

> Everything in the universe, which includes everything that makes up our being, is energy. That energy may take different forms, but whatever the form, whether it be a physical condition, a mental conflict, an emotional joy, or a spiritual realisation, is energy. When there is disharmony within us we may get a bad cough, feel angry, get a pain in our back or become disorientated and confused. If we bring together the psychological and the physical, then we can understand that there is no difference, whatever the mode of expression may be: the underlying imbalance is simply energy needing an outlet.

Each part of the body has its own unique function and purpose, and that function corresponds to an aspect of our personality (for instance, our legs are where we express our ability to move, and the direction of that movement). As we experience negativity, the energy associated to that negativity then weakens the area of the body that reflects it, leaving it vulnerable and susceptible to damage or illness. The thought will literally unease the area, thereby causing disease. 'What we put out in thought will always come back and land in the same area where we tightened at that moment,' said Reshad Feild in *Here to Heal*. By understanding the language our bodies are using as they try to tell us what is wrong, we can see the negative thought patterns and attitudes that are being expressed, and we can begin to open ourselves to more positive ones. That will then strengthen the related part of the body, enabling it to build resistance and to begin to heal.

For instance, the hands correspond to how we are handling our lives, feelings about how we are being handled, our ability to cope, as well as our ability to create and to express ourselves. When we have a problem in our hands we can therefore look to these aspects of our inner being and see where the conflict lies. If we continue putting out the same thought and tightening in the same area, then the damage will slowly increase. When we can recognise the messages, then we can connect with and help release the source of the problem. 'Many patients already know something of this link and only require an open-minded doctor to be able to use the knowledge,' wrote Dr Bernie Siegel in *Love, Medicine and Miracles*. 'As one said, "I was always considered spineless and here I've developed multiple myeloma of my backbone." A multiple sclerosis patient whose husband left her with five young children to care for, lost the use of her right hand. She had just lost her right-hand man.' By paying attention to and integrating what the body is saying, there can be a deep reconnecting with our inner needs, conflicts, confusions and feelings, all of which are not being openly expressed or even acknowledged and are therefore finding expression through the body. Bringing awareness to the part of ourselves that has been ignored or isolated is in itself a healing. It is a wonderful opportunity for change, as our bodies provide us with all the tools we need in order to understand ourselves more deeply.

Illness can lead us to a deeper appreciation of our purpose and reason for being here, for we can no longer take everything for granted. During severe or life-threatening illnesses we are confronted by our vulnerability and impermanence, by the fact that life at some point has to end. And we experience the reality that we are not alone in our pain. If we can openly accept and integrate this reality then we can begin to live in the present, free of fear. Then there is beauty where once there was ugliness, compassion and love where once there was bitterness or envy; for life becomes truly precious, to be enjoyed and lived fully. Like a flower that grows through solid concrete, our inner life force has only one desire: to reach fulfilment. It uses every method it can to show us what we need to do to enable this to happen. Confronting death is one aspect of this, as it means confronting a level of reality we rarely have to deal with.

Every cell in our bodies is aware of every other cell: each one has full intelligence of all the others. This includes all aspects of our brain that determine our emotional and mental states, as well as our memories and unconscious. Consequently, every cell in our physical bodies is in constant communication with our thoughts, emotions, desires, beliefs and self-images. As Deepak Chopra put it in *Healers on Healing,*

> Once we see ourselves as creations of intelligence, then we must admit that we are self-created. Actually, we are in the process of self-creating, because intelligence never ceases to communicate with itself. The blood is not a chemical soup; it is a multi-lane freeway in which thousands of messages, conveyed by hormones, neuropeptides, immune cells, and enzymes, are forever travelling, each intent on a mission, each capable of maintaining its own integrity as an impulse of intelligence.

The language the bodymind uses is surprisingly simple to understand. Unearthing the inner conflict is the first step; dealing with that inner conflict and transforming it from conflict to resolution and peace is what enables healing to take place. It is not an easy task, however, not one that everyone will want to undertake, for it demands that we deal with all those aspects of ourselves that we have been spending many years ignoring!

CHAPTER 2

Decoding the Language

In every created thing on earth there is an internal and an external; one of these is not given without the other, as there is no effect without a cause. . . . The external is estimated from the internal, and not the reverse. EMANUEL SWEDENBORG

As the outer expressions of our being are a direct reflection of our inner experiences; so it is our reaction or response to the events in our lives, and not the events themselves, that create our reality. What is it that is actually happening, when for instance we get an ache in our shoulder, trip over and scrape our knees, have a recurring backache or get indigestion easily? If we casually glance at all the physical ailments from which we suffer, they don't usually make much sense. But if they are looked at with the attitude that our bodies are trying to give us a message, and if we learn the language that is being used, a meaning does emerge. We can then begin to see the many subtle and delicate ways in which we are being shown what is happening within us.

Nature is never haphazard; there is always the most intricate order at work, and we are an integral part of that order. Our bodies clearly reflect the imbalances of energy within us, for when we do not recognise what is taking place psychologically or emotionally, when we are blind to our own attitudes and behaviour, then that energy will find another way to come to our attention. Physical discomfort is the last resort; we do not, after all, really want to hurt ourselves or be in pain. When physical problems emerge it is therefore time to heed the body's warning.

As the body reflects what is happening on both the conscious and unconscious levels, so the mind uses the body to express itself. It uses particular symbols and patterns with which to communicate, and these patterns manifest themselves through illnesses, diseases or accidents. By learning the language that is being used we can understand what is being communicated. In this way we have access to our own inner healing and can bring about a state of resolution. This chapter will explore in detail the various patterns and how to understand and interpret the language. Each pattern will be dealt with separately, and then in the following chapters all the symbols and understanding will be brought together to see how they apply to physical difficulties.

The Principle of Correspondences

The principle of correspondences was developed by Robert St John, founder of Metamorphosis, and is based on the 'Doctrine of Correspondences' formulated by the Swedish religious teacher Emanuel Swedenborg. It proposes that every natural physical manifestation has a relationship to a corresponding non-physical state of being or principle. A close relationship between spiritual qualities and material forms can thus be inferred, the former being archetypes of the latter. This becomes particularly clear when we study the human body and see the three primary ways in which the cells are formed: as hard tissue, soft tissue and fluids. We can then refer to the relationship that these three cell structures have with our spiritual, mental and emotional energies.

Hard Tissue

The hard tissue (primarily the bones) forms the framework upon which our body is built, like the layers of rock in the depths of the earth. It is the underlying factor without which there can be no life – the innermost central core of our physical being.

After conception, the spine is the first part of the body to develop, followed by the rest of the skeleton. The bones therefore represent that initial urge to incarnate, for if there is to be life it must have a form. The bone structure provides that form. 'Our bones', wrote Robert St John, 'portray the primary pattern of that with which we started life at conception . . . containing the inherited traits, the karmic patterns and all the other factors which are imposed upon or drawn into the new life. The spine is the centre of this structure.' As our bones correspond to our willingness-to-be (the desire for life) they enable us to manifest and move forwards into life, through the use of the muscles and fluids.

Although bones appear to be very slow-moving and lacking the energy or vibration of the rest of our tissue structure, the opposite is actually true. This hard tissue structure within us contains the most condensed form of energy. A diamond is an apt analogy. Diamonds are the hardest of crystals, meaning they are the most condensed form of matter and therefore the most energised. The harder the form, the higher the amount of atomic energy contained. So the bones represent the crystalline energy within us, that which is the densest and the most solid, yet also the most energetic, the core energy that supports life and enables it to manifest.

Just as the bones are the underlying structure which motivates the flesh and the fluids, so our spiritual energy gives life to our thoughts and feelings and is the underlying energy that speaks through our mental images, communication and emotions. Our spiritual understanding is constantly influencing our mental and emotional expression; dependent on our spirituality is our whole outlook on life, our motivation and direction. And just as there cannot be a body without bones, so we are not truly alive without being in touch with the spiritual aspect of our nature. The correspondence here is therefore between the hard tissue and our spiritual being.

A break or other trauma in the hard tissue system can thus indicate a conflict at the deepest core level within us, so deep that it hinders, if not completely stops, our movement forward on both the inner and outer levels. A break in the core energy implies a complete breakdown in communication; our inner conflict has become so great that we cannot continue as we are – we have to stop or be stopped. Then we can reassess, change direction, or see what it is within us that is in so much pain. It is a cry for help, for affection and attention, a cry that begs to be dependent on others as we invariably cannot manage on our own while we are recovering. I have often seen this in the elderly living alone who fall and break a bone. The broken bone brings them attention and company, easing the loneliness; it can even be a way of alerting relatives that to continue living alone in this way is no longer appropriate and a complete change is needed.

A break in the hard tissue can also be a break or conflict in our spiritual energy, and this affects every aspect of our being. Here the implication is that our spiritual direction or motivation is experiencing such turmoil or confusion that it cannot continue in its present state; the very depth of our being is in conflict. The part of the body where the break takes place will indicate further information about the nature of the conflict being expressed.

Soft Tissue

This comprises the flesh, fat, muscles, nerves, skin and organs. It is the tissue structure most responsible for our body shape, size, appearance and strength, for nerve equilibrium and normal functioning. Our soft tissue corresponds directly to our mental energy – as we think, so we become – and thereby expresses the continual movement of change within ourselves. The muscles provide the means for the bones, the hard tissue structure, to move and change us, in accordance with our insights and understandings.

Our soft tissue formation reflects our past experiences, our attitudes and our patterns of behaviour. Just as rigid tendons indicate rigid tendencies, so we can find past traumas and conflicts buried deep in the soft tissue. We build layers of fat to protect painful memories; we have over – or under-developed muscles that portray particular weaknesses and indulgences; tense muscles, tumours or fatty deposits imply the holding of thought patterns relating to the part of the body involved. Stiff or rigid muscles indicate stiff or rigid thought patterns, like a stiff neck that stops us from being able to move our head around to see on all sides. Instead we become locked into seeing only our own viewpoint, the one right in front of us. 'I have come to see that emotional experiences, psychological choices, and personal attitudes and images not only affect the functioning of the human organism but also strongly influence the way it is shaped and structured,' wrote Ken Dytchwald in *Bodymind.*

As the soft tissue reflects our attitudes, behaviour, experiences and hidden mental patterns, so we can look to it as a barometer, a way of measuring where we are at in ourselves. We can see how our soft tissue expresses the movement within us, as well as our conflicts and confusions. For instance, if we are experiencing a negative or painful situation then related muscles will be simultaneously tensing or twisting. They eventually become knotted or sprained and cannot be fully released until we are prepared to experience all the stored up pain that the situation contains. In the same way, when we bruise our legs the message is that we are mentally resisting the direction we are taking; peeling skin may be a shedding of old mental thought patterns or impressions that no longer fit us; when we lose excess weight we are dropping layers of protection and allowing ourselves to become open and vulnerable. The soft tissue is like the earth – it is the very substance from which our life can grow and blossom.

Fluids

Over 90 per cent of the human body is liquid: water, blood, urine, lymph, perspiration, saliva, tears, lactation, endocrine and sexual secretions. Fluids bathe our entire being and are like a great ocean moving within us, the tides flowing with our desires, feelings and impulses. As these fluids flow through and around the body, they bring with them essential nutrients and hormones (chemical messages from the brain) as well as oxygen; they also remove and dispose of waste products. But this is a very technical image. What the fluids also do is create excitement, warmth and energy, as when our lips, nipples and genitals become suffused with blood, we feel loving and excited and we want to share that with another person. Equally, our face will flush in an embarrassing situation; we become hot and red when feeling angry, or cold and white with rage when the emotion – the blood – is constricted.

In this way we can recognise how the fluids correspond to all our various emotions. As Alexander Lowen says in *Bioenergetics:* 'Sensations, feelings and emotions are the perceptions of internal movements within the relatively fluid body.' We see how phrases such as 'boiling mad' or 'hot under the collar' relate directly to the fluids responding to our emotional states; tears are a wonderful expression of our emotional energy pouring over with feeling. The heart has long been associated with love, as it is universally recognised as the symbol and centre of our passion, as well as, on a higher level, our compassion. The blood, as the circulation of that heart energy throughout the body, is the expression of both our love and all the confusing emotions related to love, as it circulates throughout ourselves and our world. Problems with the heart indicate a self-centredness and conflict with expressing or feeling love. Hardened arteries can indicate a resistance to and hardening of our emotional energies, minimising the amount of emotional expression. Urination is a release of emotions we no longer need; urinary problems therefore indicate that we are not expressing those negative emotions that should normally be released. Rather we are holding on to them, and in so doing they cause irritation and pain, as in cystitis.

Each fluid in the body corresponds to a different aspect of our emotional nature. An imbalance in the fluid system resulting in swelling, difficulty with urination, excessive bleeding or the inability to clot, sweating or excess dryness, or high blood pressure, indicates an imbalance in our emotional body, in the expression or repression of our feelings and responses. Which emotion it is will depend on which fluid is being affected (see Chapter 6).

The fluids give direction and purpose to the movement that is possible through the bones and muscles. In the same way our emotions express our spiritual intent, the power and ecstasy of that energy; and they give direction and purpose to our mental energy.

Left and Right Sides

Although we usually think of ourselves as well balanced, particularly one side to the other, there are some very important differences. The two sides of the body represent the two sides of the brain, each side being responsible for quite different functions.

The Right Side

The left side of the brain actually controls the right side of the body. This aspect of our being, in both men and women, represents the masculine nature: the intellectual, aggressive, and assertive, that which deals with daily reality, practical and work issues, is authoritative, logical and rational. This is known as the Yang nature, the part of us that we tend to use most. It reflects our relationship to our masculine nature, whether that be within ourselves, in our relationships, or with masculine figures in our lives such as our father, son, husband or boyfriend. In men, problems of this side of the body can represent the conflict of competition, or issues of masculinity. In women, this side tends to reflect conflicts such as the difficulty of being a career woman and integrating a more masculine, assertive nature into the stereotype of the feminine. For instance, Ellie came to see me experiencing slight numbness in the whole right side of her body, something she had felt since she was a teenager. She had been a tomboy all her childhood, and as we talked she now realised that the numbness had developed in response to her father's desire that she become a young lady at puberty and train as a secretary, when what she really wanted to do was to become a fighter pilot! Out of respect for her father she cut off her more aggressive responses, or rather she withdrew feeling from that aspect of her personality, thereby creating a rejected and cold (numb) feeling in that part of her that represented her assertiveness (the right side). In denying this aspect of her personality she was able to do what her father wanted without resentment. For Ellie, the healing involved forgiving her father for imposing his wishes on her, developing the confidence to do what she really wanted to, for her own sake, and forgiving herself for having repressed her feelings. It meant bringing the repressed and unacknowledged part of her being back to life.

The Left Side

The right side of the brain connects with the left side of the body and represents the feminine principle, or Yin energy. This is our creative and artistic nature, the gentle, receptive, irrational and intuitive – the inner world. It is the side that many of us are either out of touch with or are unsure how to express. It represents our relationship to the feminine nature, both within ourselves and with others. Difficulties on the left side in a man can indicate conflict with expressing his caring and nurturing qualities, his ability to cry or to comfort. It can also show a difficulty in receiving, especially love or emotional release. In women it can indicate confusion with expressing femininity, or conflict with being a woman and meeting up to the expectations of what a woman should be. In both sexes it can relate directly to relationships with women – for instance to our mother, daughter, wife or girlfriend.

Centres of Activity

We have one main centre of activity: the head. From here all action starts as thought, and is then reflected through our two primary means of expression: the moving centre and the doing centre.

The physical development of the embryo, shortly after conception, starts with the formation of the head and the spine (see p.28). It is a downward movement of energy, known as cephalo-caudal development. This energy then moves outwards from that central force into the legs and arms (into moving and doing). This is known as proxi-modistal development. 'If consciousness depends to any extent upon the development of the physical body as the vessel of consciousness,' wrote Jonathan Damian in *Wholistic Phenomenology*, 'then the consciousness of the embryo proceeds from an enclosed "centre", outwards to the more exposed extremities.' In exploring the moving and doing centres we will be focusing on our psychological and emotional relationship to the inner and outer expressions of these primary areas.

The Moving Centre

From the hips down to our feet is our moving centre, representing the direction we are taking, the progression of our lives in relation to our environment, and the movement we are making within ourselves. This latter aspect relates directly to the pelvis which represents our inner direction and our deepest feelings and thoughts, our conflicts or ease, about our personal movement. The pelvis is the area where we can give birth physically to new life and psychologically to new movement within ourselves; from here we can move upwards to new areas of understanding as we expand our consciousness, (see chapter 3) or downwards as we move into the world through the feet. The pelvis also expresses the polarity of our movement in relation to the movement of others, for this is the area of communication and external involvement. It is where we can express our heart energy through the sharing of our sexuality, and the release of fear and anger through urination; it corresponds to our social, more outward aspects, those which are found in our relationships.

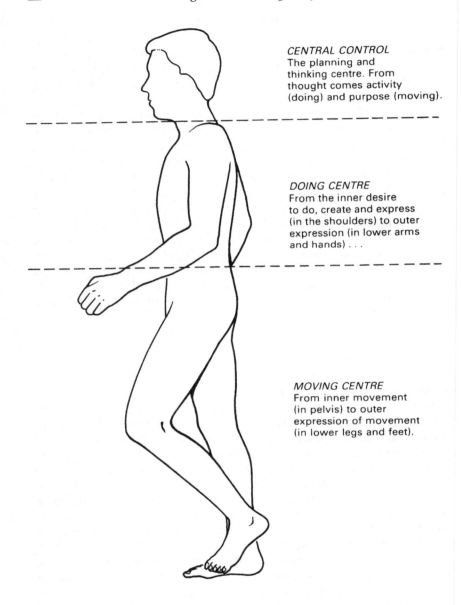

Fig.1 Centres of Activity

The pelvis reflects the movement we are taking within ourselves, so as the energy moves down the legs it begins to emerge into the world; from being an inward movement it becomes externalised. Our legs therefore express our feelings and attitudes about our movement. For instance, our knees are where we kneel, and kneeling is the acknowledgement of higher authority or power through surrender and humility. The knees are also our shock absorbers, giving grace to our movement over what is often a rough terrain. Problems in this area might relate to self-assurance, pride and obstinacy; or it may be that the terrain we are crossing is proving too hard for us to be able to continue. Such qualities hinder our movement forward.

Our ankles represent our mental or spiritual support system, that which we rely and depend on as the foundation of our activity. If an ankle gives way then the whole body collapses, we fall, and our movement forward is halted. This indicates a collapse in our support system, in that which has been holding us up, implying that the direction in which we were going needs to be reassessed or changed.

Our feet represent the direction we are taking in the world. They are our contact with mother earth and through them we have standing and strength in our place in the world. Our feet go forward first and furthest, so they represent our most external movement and direction. They also reflect within them every aspect of our being as it is responding to that movement. When the movement or direction is in conflict with our inner desires, then we may hurt our feet in some way, or stub a toe.

The moving centre is that part of the body, from the pelvis downwards, that is to do with stabilising, balancing, supporting, being grounded and rooted in the world. When this lower half of the body is proportionately larger than the top half, it suggests that we are extremely well-grounded and 'at home' in the world, but may be out of touch with our more private feelings, and with our ability to contact or express these, as if they are being constricted inside. When the lower half is proportionately smaller than the top half, it indicates a lack of connection with the earth – there is insufficient energy moving down through the body and reaching the ground. It would suggest that emphasis is being placed on the effect we are having in the world, on 'putting up a big front', rather than in being solid and grounded in our standing. This implies that, although we can easily express ourselves, we have nowhere to put the feelings, so they have no solid foundation.

The Doing Centre

From the spine across the shoulders and down to the hands is our doing centre: how we feel about what we are doing, about what is being done to us, about our capability to handle our lives. This area also represents our desire to express ourselves: through the use of our hands we can express our innermost artistic and creative energies; through our arms and hands we can share our love and giving energy from the heart; through caressing, touching and holding we can reach out, pull in or push away.

The shoulders express this on the inner levels – specifically our deeply personal feelings about what we are doing, or what is being done to us. How many of us are really doing what we want to do? How often do we wish we could undo something already done? And how often are we in real conflict about what we should be doing? It is here that we carry our burdens, begrudgingly doing something even if we don't really want to, or holding on to guilt and negative emotions from the past to do with something we have already done. A 'cold shoulder' can be an emotional cold we are experiencing within ourselves towards someone or something, or it may be a cold shoulder being directed towards us from someone else.

The arms move this doing energy outwards, from our inner feelings and desires to their expression in the world. The elbows give flexibility and grace to this flow of energy, adding the necessary effort to ensure manifestation. The wrists move it out further. A conflict in the wrist can indicate there is something we should be, or want to be doing but are not; for some reason we are holding back from that final expression.

By the time we reach the hands, the expression is one of how we think or feel about what we are doing out in the world; here we hold on to events or feelings, or are unable to grasp new situations. The hands are our means for creative release; through them we communicate and share. As they are the most outward expression of our doing energy, so we often push them out too far, try to do too much, or feel confused about what we are doing. Our hands then get hurt, or we burn or cut a finger.

The Pre-natal Pattern

This pattern traces the development of consciousness that takes place during the gestation period, from pre-conception to birth, and how this development is reflected in the body. The pre-natal pattern has been most extensively understood in the work of Metamorphosis, which recognises not only that this time period is accessible through various parts of the body, but that we can instigate deep change by working with these specific areas. Readers who wish to study this further should read *The Metamorphic Technique* (see Bibliography).

We already know that the moment of conception sets in matter all the genetic inheritances that are going to form us. The genes are like the building bricks of our being; the blueprint that is formed at conception is built with these bricks throughout the gestation period. But can we honestly say that genes make up the whole of us, that genes create that which is uniquely us? Can genes form consciousness, thoughts, creativity, feelings, ideas, insights?

This pre-natal pattern is based on the presumption that at the moment of conception there is an energy present apart from the sperm and ova. This energy is the incoming being-to-be. There are many names and a variety of spiritual thoughts surrounding this, all tending to imply that the new being first emerges totally in the abstract, as consciousness without form; it is then attracted towards the physical plane, and is further attracted to two particular people within that physical plane, much as a magnet attracts. As conception takes place, the being-to-be enters into matter. As gestation progresses, all the individual potentials and characteristics of that being-to-be are built into and established within it. Everything that occurs during the gestation period and beyond is therefore a part of that which we attracted to us at conception.

The growth of the foetus from a single cell to a fully formed human being is an extraordinary process of creation, encompassing not only physical development but also the development of consciousness. Here we are primarily concerned with the relationship between our bodies and the changes in consciousness we experienced as a foetus, for these changes are not only mirrored in our bodies but are constantly influencing us. These different states of consciousness also create a specific language used by the mind to express certain states of being.

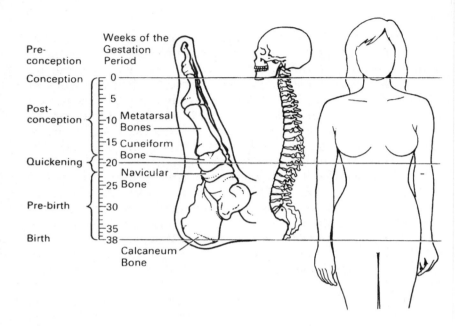

Fig.2 Chart of the Pre-natal Pattern as formulated by Robert St John

The gestation pattern can be accessed through the spinal reflexes in the feet, hands and head, and on the spine itself (these are the areas used in the Metamorphic Technique). Its relationship to the spine can be seen in Fig. 2. We will work our way through the specific stages of the gestation period from conception to post-conception, quickening, pre-birth and birth. We shall then look at pre-conception in the light of our new understanding.

Conception

This is a focal moment in time, an explosion of energies as the sperm and ova meet and merge their individual identities into one, creating the potential physical structure of the new being. It is the time when all the factors or influences that are going to make 'us' are brought together: the genetic inheritance, the race, time, location and condition of our lives to be. All these coalesce, each one adding a particular flavour to the whole, thereby forming the blueprint of the being-to-be.

At conception all the genetic inheritances we shall manifest in our lives, such as the colour of our hair or a special character trait, are present; in the same way our 'non-genetic' inheritances are also present – those factors that are unique to us and that form our specific path. For instance, even our astrological sign appears to be defined at this very early stage. As there are physical characteristics attributed to each astrological sign and our physical being is formed during early gestation, it would appear that at conception we have already attracted the zodiac sign we are going to be born with. When we then come under the influence of the pre-chosen star formation, so the stimulus to be born arises. An article in *Newsweek* by Walter Goodman on August 30th 1982, stated,

> The unborn child tends to initiate its own birth process in response to a particular planetary configuration. In this mysterious process, the planets are somehow acting as celestial midwives. Some kind of signal emanating from the planets may somehow interact with the foetus in the womb, stimulating it to struggle into birth at a certain time. . . . Perhaps it is not the moment of birth that selects the future, but rather the future that selects the moment of birth.

The potential for everything we are going to be in this world thus appears to be present at the moment of conception and is built into our being as the gestation period develops. The reality of that potential manifesting in life is then determined by our level of awareness and how we choose to live our lives. The seeds are all present at conception; how they grow depends upon the amount of gardening and watering we are prepared to do.

There are many theories as to when the consciousness of the new being enters the cell structure, but it seems that from the moment of conception there is a conscious awareness, a guiding intelligence that is present. There are many names for this in-coming energy: the soul, spirit, the life force. In essence it is intelligence, pure and very purposeful in its intent. That pure intelligence is the consciousness of the new being. Conception is the moment when this energy moves from a formless state into form, giving the single cell its life.

Conception is the bridge between the absolute and the relative, between that which is beyond time, space and matter, and that which is in time, space and matter. Crossing this bridge demands a commitment to being here and to participating fully in life. The physical correspondence to conception is the neck, and here we can see a direct relationship as the neck is the bridge between the abstract (the head) and the physical reality (the body). Breath and food that we take in through the head have to pass through the neck to get to the body in order to maintain our physical existence; in the same way thoughts and feelings from the head will manifest in the body, giving it movement and purpose. Just as with the conception of any new idea or project, there has to be a manifestation into the physical form for that idea to become a reality. In this way, from conception comes the rest of gestation, or from the neck comes the rest of the body. The neck represents the in-taking, the beginning of life. It is here that we swallow the reality that then forms the essence of our being.

The neck is extremely vulnerable, especially as a cut-off point between the mind and the body. For instance, we may feel a disgust or abhorrence of our bodies, perhaps due to having come into a situation that rejected us immediately, such as being conceived during a rape or being a 'mistake'. In which case we will ignore or reject our physical presence in the same way as we were rejected at that moment of conception. If we are particularly cerebral, if our main energy resides in our heads and we are not especially physical or aware of our bodies, then we are most likely to manifest difficulties in the neck area, such as tension or arthritis. It is as if we have never really entered into our bodies – there is no real feeling or knowledge about our physical existence, no direct experience of how it works or what it needs. As conception is the point of coming into matter we might have come in reluctantly, preferring to stay in the absolute rather than to come in to relative reality! Problems in the neck area can arise because the energy is not flowing freely due to this mindbody separation, and to a lack of commitment to being here in the world.

Post-conception

Within a very short time after conception, the single cell has not only divided many times over but has also travelled into the womb and made its home there. It then begins to change shape and to elongate, forming what is called the 'Primordial Streak', which is the first growth of the head and spine. As the foetus develops, it goes on to resemble all other forms of animal life, eventually emerging as a human. This process is described as 'ontogeny recapitulating phylogeny'. In other words, we have within us all of creation, and we pass through the whole process of evolution to reach our human form. This in itself shows us how we are truly one with all life!

Post-conception consists of the first four and a half months of the gestation period, during which time the foetus is primarily focused only on itself and its development. It is barely moving, so it has not yet encountered the fact that there is anyone or anything else present other than itself. The foetus does not distinguish between itself and its environment – in its mind there is only one, and everything in the universe is an aspect of that one. This is an extremely inward time, a period of intense development within the foetus, the forming of the individual. To quote *The Metamorphic Technique*,

> The word individual comes from the Latin, *'individuus'*, i.e. without division. In this sense, the *true* individual experiences no division, is totally at one with everything else. So here, the new life, whilst forming itself as a separate being, simultaneously knows no difference between itself and its environment. This can be seen in a paradoxical way, as an unawareness of personal individuality, and as an awareness of true individuality.

This time of development corresponds to the development on the inner levels, where there is no connection with or awareness of anything existing beyond self. It is the relationship between myself and I. Post-conception physically corresponds to the chest, from the neck to the solar plexus. Therefore all the organs and areas of the body that fall into this chest area have a connection to this inward aspect of consciousness; difficulties here will basically be indicating a problem with our inner world, our feelings, under-standing and concept of ourselves, as compared to a difficulty with relationships or between ourselves and our world. Problems can indicate a dislike for or anger with ourselves, a self-centred-ness, or an inability to share ourselves with others, thereby becoming locked into our own introverted world-view.

The heart, for instance, has long been seen as the seat of love within us, as the symbol of our love centre. From here, the love goes out to our world, symbolised by the bloodstream circulating throughout our body. The heart is in the chest, so a problem in the heart area is an indication of a problem not just with love, but with love for ourselves, the ability to express or share that love (through circulation), or even to feel love at all, to the point of shutting down this centre. Later we shall see how the other specifics in this region (such as the lungs) all relate to this inward, almost introvert-type energy. For this is the area of our innermost concerns: the chest representing our personal issues, where only self is present.

Quickening

This is the moment, at about four and a half months when the foetus first begins to move and explore its environment. In so doing it becomes aware that there is something else out there, separate to itself. The foetus hits something (the walls of the womb) that is not it. This is the transition from awareness of self to awareness of other than self, as well as the discovery of limitation. It is the beginning of relationship, the first awareness of and opening to the world. This moment of transition is a point of great focus, a tremendous shift in consciousness, away from self and into relationship, from one to duality.

This time corresponds to the solar plexus, to the diaphragm and the other organs in that area. This is a pivotal point between the chest, the inner part of our being, and the abdomen, the more outward expression. A physical problem here therefore tends to indicate that there is either an inability to express outwardly what is within, or an inability to contact that which is within from the outside. In other words, there is a holding back or blocking off of feelings from expression. It also indicates a separation of the private and public aspects of our nature, the place where we 'draw the line'; it represents our ability to make the transition from thought to form, from personal to relationship. If the transition cannot be made, then the energy becomes held within the upper chest and the introvert is born, unable to express himself. Then the inner world becomes very private and separate and there will be no sharing. Or the energy becomes held in the lower abdomen and the extrovert is born, unable to contact his real feelings, and the outer expression becomes shallow and lacks meaning.

Pre-birth

This is the last four and a half months of gestation, during which time the foetus, now formed, is preparing for birth. This is a time of action as the foetus explores and discovers the limitations and possibilities within its world. It is the time of developing self in relationship to and in communication with others. It is where the energy is moving outwards in response. In preparing for ultimate separation from the mother, this is also a time of defining the individual.

This period corresponds to the abdomen, from the solar plexus to the genitals. Difficulties in this area as a whole are therefore connected to our place in the world, to our relationships, communication and sense of personal standing. The abdomen represents the relationship between ourselves and the outside world, how we feel about what we are both receiving from and giving to our world, or a conflict between who we are and who the world thinks we are. The abdomen is where all the emotions, thoughts, attitudes and feelings that we have concerning our reality are absorbed, integrated or rejected, and hopefully, resolved. In *Bodymind* Ken Dytchwald says,

> The belly is the feeling centre of the bodymind. It is here within our bellies that many of our emotions and passions originate. When something is happening in our lives that gives birth to feelings, many of these emotions will 'grow' out of our guts and will then spread outward through the rest of our bodymind on whatever path is appropriate.

The intestines are where we assimilate and digest food; this is also where we assimilate and digest our reality, and our ability to communicate and cope with that reality. Pre-birth is the preparation time for relationship, and so it is in this abdominal area that we focus all our feelings and attitudes about our relationships and our world. Constipation or other digestive disorders are a direct response to our way of dealing with our reality; whereas kidney or bladder problems are an irritation and anger to do with expressing ourselves in our world.

Birth

This is a time of tremendous transition and lays the foundation for how we experience the world and our place in it. Birth can give us a sense of security and love, or it can be the basis for many of our adult fears and neuroses. Here the mother is most active, while at conception it was the father who was most dominant. Birth has been likened to the ultimate form of rejection by our mother, for we are being forcibly pushed into action away from her. We are emerging from a warm, dark, secure place, and if we are born into a situation of bright lights and loud noises, are held upside down and slapped, then finally separated from our mother, there is little doubt that our first impressions of the world will be that it is a cruel, aggressive, fearful and lonely place. No sense of being gently and lovingly welcomed here! Rather than experiencing the important bonding, eye contact, touching, smell and experience of mother and child that triggers many of the infant's necessary functions and creates a sense of joy and acceptance, the baby is having to armour itself against the insensitivities being perpetrated against it. As the French obstetrician Frederic Leboyer has said, 'A *person* is there, fully conscious, deserving of respect.'

Birth is the separation of mother and child as one into the world of duality, of two. It is the movement from a closed to an open state. This can create a deep level of trauma, and if the situation includes fear, panic and alienation then invariably later in life, when confronted with situations of radical change, we will react in the same way: we will be fearful, will panic, or will feel isolated and alone in our experience. If the transition was a loving and fearless one, however, then times of great change are not a difficulty and we are able to respond with courage and openness. If we were born by caesarian section we may find, when confronted with change at a later time, that we can see the other side, know that we can get there but have no idea how; we would rather just sit back and wait for it to be over. Our experience of transition was that someone else did it for us. If we were born drugged we will tend to respond to times of change later in life by blanking out; we will be unaware of what change means for there is no conscious experience of transition to refer to.

Birth is therefore a moment of shifting from inner to outer, from darkness to light. This shift in consciousness affects our later response to transition, it colours our desire for change and our ability to move from one place in ourselves to another, to let go of the past and move into the present.

The birth area, the pelvis, is the area where we can give birth not just physically but also to ourselves psychologically – in other words be able to become a true individual within our world. It represents our ability to move on within ourselves, to develop new aspects and to bring them to life. It represents completion, yet it is also a new beginning. As we shall see later, there are other factors that add to this being an area of beginning, of new direction and movement, but the quality of that movement will be highly coloured by the emotions and factors present at the birth itself.

Pre-conception

We can now take this pattern of gestation – from conception through the development of self, the development of relationship, to the emergence into an expanded environment – and apply it to the time before conception, to pre-conception. Here the pattern is reversed, as we move from the fully open and limitless space of the infinite (pre-conception) to the limited physical world of conception.

Pre-conception cannot be defined in terms of time, space and matter as it is prior to the moment of materialisation at conception. However, the mystical teachings all speak of this period with a reverence and authority gained through insight and experience. Pre-conception is when the intelligence of the being-to-be is first moving from the abstract towards the relative, but it is still in the abstract. The impulse to incarnate and come into being is therefore seen as starting before conception; and here it appears that there is an abstract gestation pattern, a pattern very similar to the physical one outlined above.

Energy is vibration, and in order for it to manifest physically it has to vibrate at a denser, slower rate than it does in the abstract. An analogy with an electrical generator and a light bulb can help explain this. Although the light bulb uses electricity, it cannot be plugged straight into a generator for the power would be too great and the light bulb would explode. The electricity has to be slowed down until it emerges at a rate that the light bulb can use. The electricity is the same, simply moving at a denser or slower vibrational rate. In a similar way formless, infinite energy has to slow down in order to emerge and appear as form.

Physical conception corresponds to the moment when the being-to-be emerges into physical life. Abstract conception corresponds to the moment when intelligence, as vibration, emerges from the formless. It is the first movement of energy away from the infinite towards the finite. This is the beginning of a new creation cycle; a shift of energy away from the purely abstract towards the concept of formation, indicating the first slowing of the vibrational rate.

During physical gestation the post-conception stage is one of inner development and of oneness with the surrounding environment, with no awareness of other than one. With the abstract post-conception stage we find a defining of the energy within the continuum of the infinite, just as a drop of water from a pool is still water, despite having been separated from the whole. The energy is in a state of pure abstract oneness; awareness of form, duality or separation has not yet developed.

The quickening point in the physical gestation is like a pivot between the inner and the outer energies as consciousness becomes aware of other than one. In the same way, abstract

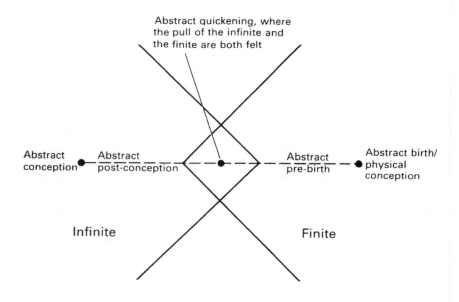

Fig.3 The Abstract Gestation/Pre-conception, as intelligence moves from the infinite toward the finite.

gestation marks a pivotal moment of moving away from the abstract towards the relative. It is a second slowing of the vibrational rate as intelligence becomes more clearly focused on matter. Here it is beginning to turn away from the infinite and to turn towards the finite, just as our physical quickening represents a movement from oneness to relationship. The shift in awareness is towards the denser manifestation of matter and is a defining of direction.

The abstract pre-birth further defines this movement towards form. Intelligence is responding to the pull of the physical plane and all the implications that this plane involves, in contrast to the formless. During the abstract pre-birth stage there is a growing awareness of what is approaching and a preparation for the coming change, just as in the physical pre-birth stage there is a preparation for relationship.

The birth point of the abstract gestation corresponds to conception on the physical level. It is the merging of the incoming intelligence with the vibrational rates of the parents-to-be. This is the final slowing down of the vibrational rate in order for consciousness to enter matter. Energy from the generator is now usable in the light bulb. Having left the infinite behind, the focus is solely on development in the physical plane.

This pre-conception period corresponds to the head. In this way we can see how the head is the centre for mystical, abstract and even spiritual energy. Thought is the precursor of action, just as energy is the precursor of the physical form. The head is the creative centre, the focal point for the most profound aspects of our nature, as well as being the manifestation of pure intelligence. Problems to do with the head are therefore related to the more formless and spiritual aspects of our being.

Consciousness evolves in the abstract, moving through particular stages as it gravitates towards conception. Once it has merged with the physical factors necessary to create life it then develops in a pattern similar to the one it has just experienced, this time adapting to all the factors in the physical realm of existence. We see this pattern repeated again with life, as from birth we go through an intensely inward time, the first fifteen or twenty years being totally 'I' centred with the development of the individual. This is then followed by transition to a state of relationship and awareness of the world as we become adults. From here we go through yet another transition and, in dying, are born into a new realm. In every birth there is a death: the death of the mother and child as one, as it is born into the birth of two. In every death there is also a birth: the birth of the infinite out of one, of limitlessness out of individuality.

The Endocrine System

This pattern is somewhat more complex than the previous ones, and certainly less obvious. It is often linked to the chakra system, which is outlined in chapter 3.

Here we shall not be making a scientific study of endocrinology but looking at the endocrine glands from a more metaphysical and philosophical viewpoint, connecting them to the gestation pattern development as seen above, to the stepping down of energy into the physical world. Interestingly, the word 'endocrinology' is derived from the Greek words meaning 'within' and 'I separately', and this clearly portrays the role it plays in our lives. The endocrine glands are distinguished from other glands by the fact that their secretions are of such power and strength that they maintain a specific equilibrium

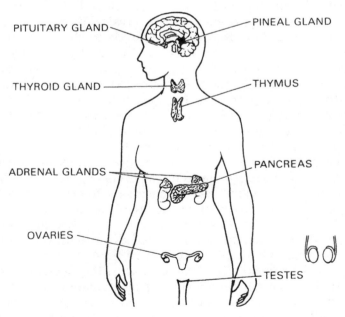

PITUITARY GLAND

PINEAL GLAND

THYROID GLAND

THYMUS

ADRENAL GLANDS

PANCREAS

OVARIES

TESTES

Fig.4 The Endocrine System

throughout the whole body. If the glands are in a sluggish or diseased state they will influence our outlook on life, particularly our moods, behaviour and ability to cope. We can feel depressed, become angry, or pessimistic; or we can be happy and peaceful, feel confident and optimistic – all depending on their condition.

The Pineal Gland

This small gland, situated in the mid-brain, has baffled scientists for it appears somewhat defunct. In ancient man it was apparently far larger and has since shrunk to a very small size. Its relevance can initially be seen in the fact that in normal mental conditions there are calcium crystals present, whereas in subnormal mental states these crystals are diminished or non-existent.

The pineal is also very involved in the perception of light. It produces a molecular structure called melanin that can actually translate one form of energy into another, i.e. sound waves into light waves. It can transfer energy through it without a loss of energy, acting as the interface between wave form and the particle world of matter. As Dr Joseph Chiltern Pierce has said, 'Melanin is a key molecule that, among other things, may be the link between mind and matter, the medium between brain and mind, thought and reality.' Melanin saturates every living form. In humans it is found mainly in the pineal gland, the skin, the heart and the genitals.

From this we can take the implications of the pineal gland one step further and see how it actually corresponds to the highest energy within us. In a paper called *Meditations on the Endocrine Glands* Karl König states,

> The pineal gland is impregnated by eternal ideas and gives to man the possibility of formulating his own conceptions. It is an organ of thought, by means of which we learn to 'know' and thus to change eternal ideas into earthly conceptions. Here lies the reason for Descartes' statement that the pineal gland is the seat of the human soul. The pineal gland points to the land of the spirit.

Putting together above comments such as 'interface between consciousness and reality', 'giving man the possibility of forming his own conceptions' and 'points to the land of the spirit', we can begin to see the connection of the pineal gland with the purely abstract, the infinite, and even with the point of abstract conception. Although the pineal is in the head on a physical level, its connection is with the non-physical; it is the first moment in matter that registers or is associated with the non-physical aspects of the new life. The pineal represents that first movement, first slowing, as the energy moves away from the infinite towards the finite. Through the pineal we are thus connected to the infinite. In the next chapter we shall see the connection of this gland to the crown chakra through which we can experience the highest state of enlightenment, of awakened mind.

There also appears to be a metaphysical link between the pineal gland and the gonads, the sexual glands, especially as melanin is known to have some control over the sex organs. This becomes clearer if we consider how the two main functions of these glands, sexual expression and spiritual or high mental expression, rarely occur together. Invariably one is more active at a time when the other will be suppressed, as in the life of a celibate monk.

The Pituitary Gland

Lying in the brain behind the eyes, the pituitary gland is known as the leader of the endocrine orchestra; our entire physiological balance, particularly our growth, is dependent on this small gland. It monitors and maintains all aspects of our development and is intimately connected to puberty, pregnancy, fertility and other feminine issues. Its dysfunction can lead to abnormal bodily growth patterns.

It would seem that the pituitary gland takes the movement of energy described above (and on p.34) one step further. It corresponds to the second slowing of energy, the abstract quickening point, as intelligence moves closer to matter. It is the connection between spirit and earth, a slowing of the abstract energy so that physical manifestation may occur. It is an interpretation of the non-physical into a form comprehensible by the human body, as reflected in its role in our growth and bodily functioning. In this way it interfaces between the pineal, our highest spiritual impetus, and the body, the physical manifestation of that impetus. 'If the pineal points to the land of the Spirit, the pituitary points to the earth,' wrote Karl König in *Meditations on the Endocrine Glands.* 'The human soul awakes to earthly consciousness by means of this small organ.' In Chapter 3 we will also see the connection of this gland to what is known as the Third Eye chakra.

The Thyroid and Parathyroid Glands

As the pineal relates to abstract conception and the pituitary to abstract quickening, so the relationship of these two glands enables man to come into being. The third slowing down of energy takes place at the neck, the point that corresponds to abstract birth/physical conception: the entry of the being-to-be into physical matter. The thyroid and parathyroid glands lie in the neck, the parathyroid being attached to each side of the thyroid. The thyroid has a role in maintaining our metabolic rate and in breathing. For instance, when animals hibernate it is the temporary cessation of the functioning of this gland that enables the hibernation to occur.

Karl König says of the thyroid gland,

> This organ we describe as being connected with inhaling; but the connection is not with the force that makes us inhale our breath but with a much wider process of inhaling. The thyroid is the organ that makes the earthly bodily frame inhale the human soul . . . by means of which the human soul wakes up within its body.

A booklet on psychic healing also describes this area, the throat, as being the point of conception and of the forming of the human body,

> Ancients have always known that this centre [the throat] has been responsible for a human's creativity [or the creativity of a human]. . . . This particular centre of activity is the mediator for the neural impulses and the slower vibrations that make up the solid tissue within the physical body.

The thyroid is therefore the gate between the abstract and reality, and it is the breath that it regulates, for it is the breath that gives life to the body. On p.28 it was explained how the neck is the bridge, the connection between mind and body through which breath must pass. In addition, the parathyroid gland keeps the rhythm of inhaling and exhaling in balance.

As König says of this small gland: 'This rhythm gives man the equilibrium he needs for unfolding his earthly state of consciousness.'

The Thymus Gland

Located near the heart, the thymus brings us from conception into the post-conception stage. One of this gland's main functions is to transform new immune cells into what are called T-cells. These T-cells are essential for a healthy immune system, since they traverse every part of our bodies looking for foreign, potentially dangerous intruders. Helper T-cells sound the initial alarm; killer T-cells destroy cancerous and virus-infected cells; suppressor T-cells sound the retreat when the coast is clear. In other words, emerging from the heart area that is directly related to the development of self is the ability to protect self, to protect the bodily form we are manifesting, to fight and win our battles inside without having to go outside for help. As the thymus gland is closely linked to the energy of the heart, its full functioning indicates the importance of love. When we are feeling bitter, angry, hateful or despising, whether towards ourselves or another, then our ability to fight infection and disease is lowered. When we are feeling loving, compassionate, generous and at peace, then our resilience will be far greater.

The thymus is also connected to our ability to sleep. As the energy steps down into the physical realm, so sleep emphasises the concentration of energy on the development of self that is taking place in this chest area – as seen in a foetus or a young baby that sleeps a great deal during its early life.

The Adrenals

Situated above the kidneys, the adrenals correspond to the quickening point for here we find the hormone adrenalin, produced when we are confronted with a 'flight or fight' situation. Just as the quickening point in the gestation pattern is like the pivot of a see-saw between our inner and outer worlds, so adrenalin stimulates our decision for flight (to run and go inside rather than be brave and confront) or to fight (to turn outwards and confront, regardless of inner warnings). This hormone enables us to deal with otherwise debilitating and stressful emotions in ourselves and in relations to others.

The adrenals are also essential for the maintenance of blood sugar and blood pressure. This corresponds to the role of the quickening point in bridging the private and public aspects of our nature: here we find the adrenals regulating the composition and balance of the blood (the love energy) as it passes from the private (the chest) into the public part of our being (the abdomen). In keeping the blood cleansed it is often necessary for the kidneys to extract the more negative emotions, such as anger and fear, from the blood; in this way urinary system irritations can occur if there is an overwhelming amoount of negative emotional energy.

The Gonads

Found in the ovaries of the female and in the testicles of the male, these glands relate to the pre-birth and birth stages of gestation, the coming into relationship and emerging as a separate being. They ensure our continuation through reproduction, in this way keeping us attached and bound to the physical world. They are the end of our journey, our descent on to earth, the final slowing down of our vibrational rate. They are also the beginning of our ascent. From giving birth to ourselves, we can now move forward towards a greater understanding of the infinite.

The gonads represent the sharing of ourselves with others, through our sexuality. The more esoteric Eastern teachings contain many practices that use sexual energy as a means to higher understanding, such as in Tantra. Here it is recognised that the power of sexuality is very great; that power can therefore be used for truly loving and spiritual purposes, or it can be abused or misused and may then cause degeneration and disease (when we abuse the power and balance of nature we upset the ease and create dis–ease). When there is an excess amount of energy applied to participating in sexual activity, it is most likely that there will be a corresponding lack of energy applied to spiritual activities.

CHAPTER 3

The Chakras

To understand the chakra system is to understand ourselves.

SWAMI BRAHMANANDA

As seen in the last chapter in the sections on the pre-natal pattern and the endocrine glands, energy moves from conception at the head down to our birth in the genital area. It is a descent from the absolute; at each level there is a slowing of the

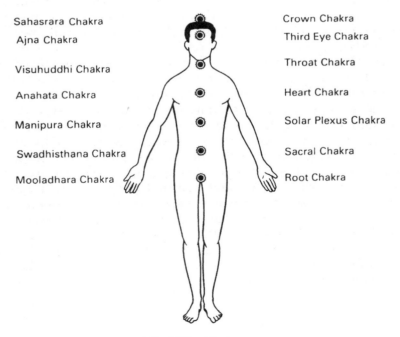

Sahasrara Chakra	Crown Chakra
Ajna Chakra	Third Eye Chakra
Visuhuddhi Chakra	Throat Chakra
Anahata Chakra	Heart Chakra
Manipura Chakra	Solar Plexus Chakra
Swadhisthana Chakra	Sacral Chakra
Mooladhara Chakra	Root Chakra

Fig.5 The Chakras

vibrational rate until we are fully in the relative world. This birth applies not just to physical birth but also symbolises the ability to give birth to new aspects of our being, whether psychologically, emotionally or spiritually. This is clearly represented by the chakra system.

All Eastern mystical teachings contain detailed references to what are called the seven chakras, or energy centres, corresponding to seven specific areas accessed through the spine. Although these chakras are not physical themselves they relate to the physical, emotional, mental and spiritual aspects of our being, directly connecting our mind and body. They are also linked to each of the glands of the endocrine system which regulate all the various functions of our being. The endocrine glands are connected to the brain and from the brain to the body. In this way the chakras act as conductors, linking the various parts of the physical body with which they are connected to the emotional or mental states associated with those parts, and with the energies of the chakras themselves. This is an example of a direct bodymind relationship.

The chakras begin at the base of the spine and move upwards. They take us from the most fundamental experiences symbolised by the sex organs to the highest, ending in enlightenment, the most supreme state of conscious experience, at the crown of the head. This crown point therefore both represents the entry of intelligence as it begins its descent (at abstract conception, the pineal gland), and is also that which 'points to the land of the spirit'. In this way we can see how the movement of the gestation pattern from conception to birth goes from awareness of self to awareness of other than self (relationship); while the movement through the chakras goes from awareness of other than self to Self awareness, the dissolving of the individual self into the cosmic Self. Each part of our body therefore represents both this downward and upward movement of energy.

Generally the higher chakras remain closed or functioning in only a minimal way. It takes conscious awareness and perseverance for them to begin to open, enabling us to reach higher states of consciousness. Exploring the chakras takes us on to a deeper level of development. Here we are looking at the more spiritual side of our nature, that which is aspiring to go beyond the mundane to a fulfilment of our highest purpose. For surely we are not here just to be born, eat, work, sleep, procreate and die? In our search to understand the bodymind language we are already entering into the world of meta-physics, of cause and effect, of the power of positive and negative thoughts and of the desire to understand hidden meanings. As we enter into the seven modes of consciousness represented by the chakras so we can take our awareness of ourselves further, to see even deeper meaning beyond that which we have already encountered.

Each chakra is symbolised by a lotus flower, and this symbolisation is very important. In order for us to grow spiritually we have to pass through three different stages, each one representing our existence on a different level of consciousness. The three are: ignorance or delusion, commitment or determination, and illumination or enlightenment. The lotus also passes through three different levels, from mud, to water, and then to air. The mud represents our ignorance, our unawareness, and this is where the lotus has its roots. It then grows through the water in its effort to reach the surface, and this is our commitment or determination to grow. Eventually the lotus reaches the air and the sunlight can enable its flower to open. This is the stage of illumination or enlightenment. The lotus is therefore a symbol of our growth from the lowest states of ignorance and delusion to the highest states of wisdom and awareness. As the flower of the lotus opens and is completely pure, free of both mud and water, so the blossoming of our true nature is pure and untainted.

Mooladhara Chakra

This first chakra, Mooladhara, which literally means 'root centre', is located in men inside and midway between the scrotum and the anus, and in women half an inch in the vagina, on the cervix. It is associated with the gonads, so this chakra is primarily to do with basic survival and primitive energy. Although 'primitive' may seem an extreme word to use, many of our present-day actions are still of this nature: fear is our most common underlying emotion, with fear about survival being a major preoccupation. The world is struggling to find enough food to feed everyone, wars rage in many different countries, we are inundated with murder, rape, pollution, materialism and unemployment. These are basically primitive activities that trigger fearful and aggressive responses.

Stress to do with survival creates not only fear but also paranoia and self-centredness, all of which affect our ability to feel grounded and at ease in our world. Much of this fear and paranoia is then expressed through our sexuality which adds guilt, shame and remorse to the list of emotions attributed to this first chakra. Stress felt here may express itself in defecation problems: when we are confronted with a life-threatening situation we can suddenly have loose bowels, or we may hold on tight and have constipation. This first chakra is involved with the exchange of primary and survival needs that easily translates into the lure of materialism and self-obsession. To deal with the energy of this chakra we need to recognise the meaninglessness of materialism and to learn to trust, to develop a giving, open and more selfless nature.

Here also at the base chakra lies the coiled serpent, the kundalini, the energy that moves upwards through the chakras to the crown, taking us from the mundane to the sublime. This chakra represents the mud from which the lotus grows, and is therefore the source of all energy. The basic condition of survival, all the fear, guilt and anxiety, is actually the ground from which we can move forwards.

Swadhisthana Chakra

This second chakra, corresponding to the reproductive and urinary systems, is located at the base of the spine. It is associated with the spleen and the pancreas, and also with the gonads. Swadhisthana means 'one's own abode or dwelling-place'. From fundamental survival issues, this chakra now connects with the energy of reproduction and excretion, bringing into action desire: sexual desire and sensory pleasure, combined with the blind urgency to hold on to those situations that give pleasure.

Balance in this chakra will be reflected in balanced sexual activity; tension or conflict will create sexual conflict which can lead to imbalance. The sexual issue is a deeply felt one and can become a dominating factor in our lives, especially since it affects many of our inter-personal relationships. In this way stress and confusion arise, for pleasure never comes without pain. That pain then gives rise to a resistance to change, an inability to be spontaneous; there is a holding on to situations as they are and a continual search for more pleasure, so as to avoid the pain. This attitude can be represented by physical problems occurring in the sexual area.

As this chakra is the seat of sexuality and basic instincts, so too it is the seat of the unconscious, a storehouse for mental impressions, the centre for man's collective and ancestral memory, that which motivates and influences our lower nature. To deal positively with the energy of this chakra is not easy, because it is so hidden within us. We have to dig deep to uncover the impressions and memories that influence us on so many levels. If we are able to do this, then, as seen earlier in this chapter, we are able to give birth to new aspects of our being, to new levels of understanding.

Manipura Chakra

As we rise above the lower levels of energy represented by the first two chakras we come to Manipura, the 'City of Jewels', also known as the fire centre. It is located at the level of the navel and the eighth thoracic vertebra and is connected to the solar plexus and the adrenals. This is the subtle centre that influences the activities of digestion and absorption of food, and the production of enzymes, particularly adrenalin.

Manipura is the beginning of our truly human qualities, as opposed to the more basic animal qualities of survival and sex. Here we emerge into the level of conscious awareness and discrimination. Manipura is the centre of power, control, status and the ego, or self-identity. From this centre our energy is concerned with whether we are liked or disliked, whether we have power or not. This is where we hold our fears and insecurities about inferiority, or we are obsessed with thinking of ourselves as the greatest and most successful. This is also the area of adrenalin – the excitement of life as well as the fear of life.

As personal power tends to be limited to our own world and does not extend to the world at large, so if our energy is fixed and functioning from this chakra we will attempt to rule or exert power, will become dominating and will try to make others conform to our own way of thinking. It is a state of ego-centredness, where there is an inability to unite or share with others and therefore we have no peace within ourselves. It is the area associated with the quickening point, to either conflict or harmony between our inner and outer worlds.

To be able to move through this chakra without becoming the slave of our own ego means developing an appreciation of and respect for others' feelings and thoughts, an acceptance that we are all different and valid in our own right. It also means being able to use our power constructively for the benefit of both ourselves and our world, rather than destructively. It is the recognition that the ego is an illusion, not a fixed means of defining who we are in the world, and therefore it has no substantial power. Physical problems in the solar plexus area can therefore relate to the conflict of power and ego-identity issues represented by this chakra; as well as the ability to take life into our being on such a level that we can fulfil our purpose for being here.

Anahata Chakra

This is the heart centre, also known as 'the space within the heart where purity resides'. It is associated with the eighth cervical vertebra, close to the thymus gland. It is here that we see the development and expression of love and affection and the higher qualities of compassion and loving kindness. Whereas the previous three chakras were predominantly to do with the world of the body, senses and mind, here we begin to move beyond, into the higher realms. This also corresponds to the post-conception stage of gestation, to the development of the individual. So here we can see the beginning of true individual experience, the higher expression of individuality, becoming free of worldly or sensual influences. It is the state of true unity with others, a recognition that we are all one.

This is the stage of developing unconditional love. Here all the lower negative emotions are transformed into empathy and selflessness, into compassion and loving kindness. It is love without expectations, without the need or desire for something in return. As John Harvey put it in *The Quiet Mind*,

> Someone functioning from the second chakra cuts a piece of chocolate cake and says, 'This is delicious! I *love* this cake!' And at the third chakra one may be possessive of another person and claim that that is love. But love as it is understood from the heart chakra has nothing to do with getting anything back, any more than the sun wants anything in return for its radiance.

It can be overwhelming to move into such a state of selflessness in what is basically a selfish world: it can create separation as others distrust our motives for being so generous or kind. Those who are on the spiritual path will recognise the inner beauty radiating outwards, but those who are not may be suspicious and paranoid – in which case a denial of these attributes can take place, a closing in of this centre. It takes great courage to become a loving and compassionate person in this world, for it is not easy to be different. But once the commitment is made, the inner joy is all-pervasive.

Vishuddhi Chakra

This chakra is associated with the cervical plexus directly behind the throat pit, at the third cervical vertebra, influencing the larynx and the thyroid gland. As seen in the pre-natal pattern, this throat area represents the bridge between the purely abstract and the relative. Vishuddhi means to purify and so here we enter into the stage of purification; here lies the ability to discriminate between the realisation and understanding that is entering our consciousness from higher levels of wisdom, and the meaningless babbling of our unconscious mind or selfish thinking. This is represented in Indian mythology by the swan with its gracefully long neck. The swan symbolises the ability to discriminate between milk and water, between truth and ignorance, between that which is skilful and that which is unskilful.

In the traditional Eastern texts this throat centre is known as the place where divine nectar is tasted. Apart from the physical occurrence of this nectar, it can also be seen symbolically as spiritual nourishment through communication and the divine word, the spoken word on the highest level. It represents a state of openness and awareness that sees how every experience is a teaching towards deeper understanding of self and self-identity. It is to do with the expression and interpretation of communication.

However, if we are shut off from receiving nourishment or love, or from being able to communicate these emotions outwardly from ourselves to another, then this centre will remain closed, causing restriction and pain. What is it that we are not being able to express fully? What emotions are getting held back in the chest? Or is it that what we are being presented with is not the promised nectar but something unsavoury and unswallowable? Is the need to be nurtured being translated as a need for food or other substances, a replacement for the truly divine love and nourishment we crave?

When the throat centre is open, the ability to speak the truth emerges. The nectar flows and the unconditional love experienced in the heart chakra finds a means of expression.

Ajna Chakra

Ajna means to command, and this chakra is known as the 'Third Eye', or 'Eye of Wisdom' centre, as it is the eye that looks inward to transcendent wisdom rather than outward to the world. Here lie knowledge and understanding of truth. The ajna chakra is associated with the brain, directly behind the centre of the eyebrows, and is connected to the pituitary gland. And just as the pituitary gland represents the stepping down of intelligence so it may manifest in form, so here the intelligence is stepping up towards infinity. The connection between this centre and the crown chakra above enables the highest knowledge to be available to man, in the same way that the pituitary gland is intimately connected to the pineal in the physical manifestation of man.

This is the chakra of the mind and of heightened self-awareness, of bliss, joy and inner vision. The ego, its self-centred way of functioning and all the confused emotions surrounding it have been left far behind. Attachment to matter and form dissolve into freedom from desire. Here the Third Eye represents the ability to 'see' all things clearly with intuitive knowledge. It is as if we are waking up from a dream, the dream of delusion that constantly clouds our perception. Now we are awake to the reality of cause and effect, to the fact that all things are dependent on each other, and we can see the subtle laws that govern man on the psychic and spiritual levels.

Sahasrara

Although technically it is not a chakra, Sahasrara is usually included as the seventh or crown chakra. Chakras exist by being within the realm of the psyche, whereas Sahasrara is beyond the psyche; it is the abode of expanded awareness. It lies at the crown of the head, corresponding to the pineal gland, that which represents the 'seat of the human soul', the gateway to pure intelligence. Here there is full awareness that there is only one, that there is no separation or duality. It is the end of individual existence, of name and form. It is the culmination and highest purpose of human existence.

This supreme experience is described by all the religious teachings, although different names may be used: nirvana, samadhi, enlightenment, communion, heaven, God, or cosmic consciousness. It is attained through unstinting effort and commitment, and by having explored and opened the previous six chakras. It is the most beautiful and blissful state of peace and oneness with all life.

Having traversed the chakra symbology, we can now see why their order is so important. We move upwards from our feet and our legs, which are like our roots, representing our ancestors and collective history; through to basic and individual survival needs, for here the individual has emerged from the collective mind, represented at the first chakra. With the second chakra comes the development of sexuality and desire; then at the third chakra we develop self-identification and personal power. This represents the end of the lower nature and the beginning of the higher nature, for in the fourth chakra comes the development of loving kindness, compassion and selflessness. It is the movement from awareness of self to awareness of other than self, a similar movement to that seen in the Pre-natal Pattern. The fifth chakra represents that of clear and divine communication; while the sixth is expanded consciousness and brilliant mind. The seventh chakra is full self-realisation or enlightenment.

CHAPTER 4

Interpretation

The world appears as a complicated tissue of events, in which connections of different kinds alternate or overlap or combine, and thereby determine the texture of the whole. ANON

THE starting point in our interpretation of the bodymind language is to first see what is physically wrong in the body. Then we look at the area where the problem is situated – whether it is in the chest, the abdomen, the legs or the arms – and the significance of that area in relation to the gestation pattern, or the moving centre or the doing centre. Is it on the right side or the left side of the body? Is it close to an endocrine gland or chakra centre? What is the nature of the tissue structure involved? Is it soft tissue that is being irritated or strained; hard tissue that has been broken; or fluids that are being released or retained? Each different aspect of the particular difficulty needs to be written down or listed, so that a complete picture can emerge.

Most importantly, how does the damaged area or illness *feel*? By entering into the sensation we can experience the emotions involved. What words do we use to describe it? Is it a certain colour, emotion, texture or temperature? Very often the inner feeling of a condition, and the words we use to describe it, will tell us a great deal about what is going on. How does it feel to be a pulled muscle? Can we feel the strain and tension in ourselves that it represents? I remember a client who had suffered from polio as a young child. He told me how, with the birth of his younger brother, he felt as if he was being left hanging emotionally by his mother. Later he remembered being in the hospital following his illness and feeling as if his body was just hanging there, lifeless and helpless. Without realising it he had used the same word twice to describe his feelings. As we explored this further he began to see what the polio had symbolised for him, and therefore what he needed to do in order to balance the emotional imprint from his childhood.

The body will be manifesting the unconscious patterns: those that are not being acknowledged or recognised consciously, but are being denied or ignored. The conscious ones we are already familiar with and we are, hopefully, dealing with them. The unconscious energies are the ones trying to make themselves known to us so that they can be released and resolved; in their isolation they are crying out for help. Consequently we each have our own way of expressing our bodymind, as we all have our own unique issues. It is therefore important to look at all the different interpretations of the language being used, for only one particular aspect may be appropriate. For instance, abnormally sweaty feet may represent a release and letting go of old emotions, but they may just as easily represent an excess of emotion not being fully acknowledged within.

To find the psychological and emotional causes of our bodymind expression, we usually need to look back six to twelve months prior to the onset of the physical difficulty. What was happening for us at that time with our family or loved ones? Was there some shock or trauma that dug deep inside us? Was there a disappointment at work? Or was there a growing feeling of anger, discontent or insecurity? Is our nature one that is constantly criticising, being resentful or playing the martyr? The mind uses the body only as a last resort to give us a message. Prior to this, the imbalance manifests on an inner level and it is here that we need to direct our attention and awareness. It means being deeply honest with ourselves, acknowledging our true feelings about a situation, even if those feelings are negative or seem inappropriate. It means looking into some of the darkest and murkiest parts of ourselves. As the energy is not being acknowledged on these inner levels, so it is having to find expression through the physical level. To free the body we have to recognise, accept and integrate the inner conflict. If we cannot find the cause in the previous year, then looking further back may be necessary.

I remember a forty-six-year-old woman, Elizabeth, coming to see me with her parents. She was suffering from a neurotic fear of metal objects, as well as from a large amount of excess weight extending from her waist to her knees. We determined that both these conditions had started twenty-three years earlier. I asked her what had happened at that time, but she could not recall anything of real significance. Unable to control herself, Elizabeth's mother finally butted in, explaining that something certainly *had* happened then. That was when Elizabeth had found out that her husband of only six weeks, the first man she had ever really loved, was actually gay. What had this meant to her? Even though she was loved as a person by her husband, it had meant a rejection of her as a woman, and especially of her sexuality. Elizabeth had completely buried this memory. That act of denial contributed directly to her excess weight, which was acting as padding around the area of her sexual expression, enabling her to continue to avoid dealing with the feelings locked inside. Her husband had been a metal worker. Elizabeth could not stand to be near metal objects.

The body may also be manifesting an inner problem that has already been resolved, as the body takes a longer time to change than the mind does. For instance, a period of intense anger might have now reached resolution and passed, but the body can still be experiencing it and reflecting it, perhaps as a liver or spleen imbalance. In these cases we simply have to look further back than the immediate past, to see what it was that so upset our system. We also need to see if we have any other hidden issues that are maintaining the symptoms or conditions, rather than letting them be released. Are we really ready and willing to be well, to be free of our limited state? Chapter 7 explores these important questions in more detail.

We may also have been told, or may believe, that our problems are due to an unresolved past life experience, something that we have brought with us into this life. This may be so. There are definitely some physical problems, especially in children, that defy rational explanation and would appear to be something that is working its way through the person. But if we use the influence of past lives as an excuse not to take any action to change the situation in this life, then we are missing the point. We are manifesting these problems *now* in order that we resolve them and let them go. We don't, after all, want to take them on into yet another life! It really doesn't matter how far back an issue goes, whether it be one year or a few hundred years: the same action is needed if we are to let go and move beyond our limitations.

In summary, the guidelines we use and can ask ourselves are:

1. What is the nature, function and part of the body affected?

2. What are the inner feelings and language being used to describe the difficulty?

3. What were the time and the conditions surrounding the onset of the symptoms?

4. What is the pay-off or hidden agenda that we may have that is keeping the situation in the present?

Once we have seen what the body is saying and we have located the inner area of repressed conflict, then we need to find the most appropriate way of enabling ourselves to release the old patterns and move into a new understanding. Chapters 7 and 8 offer suggestions and guidelines to finding the means for healing and resolution most suitable to each one of us.

CHAPTER 5

From the Head to the Toes

All that exists on earth exists in one dynamic or another in every dimension of reality beyond earth. Form is but one expression of what we see around us. That expression shifts and changes in countless ways that directly relate to the many realities which exist on all levels. There is not one thing about earth that does not exist on all other levels of reality. ANON

CHAPTERS 2 and 3 outlined the main patterns that the bodymind uses to express inner conflicts, confusions and disharmonies. Now we can start putting these patterns together so that they begin to make sense as a whole. In working our way through the bodymind in this way we are able to gain a deeper understanding of the language and how to work with it.

The Head

The head is our centre of communication, from where we meet the world through our hearing, sight, taste and smell, and the world meets us through our speech and expression. All our sensory impressions and communications take place here, for this is 'central control'. But the head is far more than just a communications centre. As seen in the gestation pattern, the head is also connected with pre-conception and the purely abstract energy that this period symbolises. Represented here is the energy as intelligence comes from the infinite towards form, and as it moves up and reconnects with the infinite. All forms of mental difficulties can thus be seen as actually being drawn towards the incoming being-to-be even before conception, as if the incoming energy is attracting particular mental states to itself as it comes towards matter. There is therefore a strong connection between our mental attributes and conflicts, and our spiritual energies.

This can be seen in the interesting fact that the head has bone – the hard tissue (or spiritual energy) – surrounding the soft tissue and fluid (the mental and emotional energies), as the skull surrounds the contents of the head. On the other hand, in the rest of the body, the bone is on the inside (the skeleton) with the soft tissue and fluids covering it. This shows how the head, representing the abstract and our connection to the infinite, is primarily spiritual, with the mental and emotional energies under or within that spiritual influence. As the energy comes into manifestation with the formation of the body, so the spiritual energy becomes less obvious; it is more discreet and goes underground, as it were, influencing the mental and emotional energies from within. The head is our centre on the highest level for all that is free of materialisation; it is where our energy comes into the physical field and slowly steps down so it may manifest itself in the world, through the pineal and pituitary glands and the central governing system. The head is therefore in the realms of the abstract. As the energy comes into matter (at the neck – conception) so it now has to operate through the physical body, through our movement and direction on earth, so it takes a more inward position.

If we suffer from a headache it is because the arteries in the head have become constricted and are causing intense pulsating pressure. Blood carries our feelings, particularly feelings to do with love and acceptance and their opposites, hate, anger and rejection. Through the arteries and veins we both give and receive love. The constriction in the head therefore tends to indicate an inability to express or receive such feelings; it is a constricting, if not an actual closing down, of expression. Allowing our feelings free expression, or receiving another's expressive emotions, is not easy because we may experience them in the head but then have to translate them through the more dense and solid body. This is how a bodymind separation can so easily develop: the body experiences one thing and the head experiences another, and we are unable to bring the two together. Tension and pressure headaches are due to the tension and pressure we put ourselves through in this process. See Chapter 6 for more information on headaches.

The head is where we withdraw to, away from the world; it is where we can develop and reach the highest levels of consciousness. From here we communicate with the physical world around us, the inner world within us, and the higher realms above us. Each part of our head represents a different aspect of this expansive communication, receiving impressions and sensations from the body and expressing them outwardly. However, when the head is separated from the body then that communication becomes blocked and stifled.

The Face

Our face is the first part of our being that greets the world; it is from here that the world will make judgments and form impressions about who we are, what sort of person we are, even whether we are likeable or not. Through our face we communicate not only how we look externally, but how we look internally: whether we are closed or open, willing to share; whether we are trustworthy or shifty and sly; and whether we are basically happy and joyful, or if we are full of sadness. It is the mask we can hide behind, or the open expression of our inner selves. The face of an enlightened being is unmistakable, as nothing is hidden, it simply radiates with inner peace; while the face of a tormented and depressed person will be furrowed, closed, dark and heavy.

We shape and form our face according to our inner nature, as well as according to who we think we are, or pretend we are. We will use expressions such as smiling or frowning either to express our real feelings, or to hide those feelings. If we are habitually hiding behind a mask then our facial muscles will become tense and distorted, taking on the mask as a real expression. Remember being told as a child not to make an ugly face in case the wind changed and then your expression would be locked forever in that position? If we make an ugly face too often, then our muscles become used to that formation and set in it. A mask may be hiding our feelings from the world as much as it may be protecting us from seeing our own real feelings. If we are hiding from others, it is usually because we do not like what we see in ourselves.

The face also refers to our image, identity or ego. As when we 'lose face', it indicates a loss of pride or ego-standing. If we have courage and inner strength then we are able to 'face up' to situations; if we do not, then we have somehow failed. A sense of incompetence or inadequacy, irritation with ourselves, criticism, self-dislike or feelings of being unloved can all result in the facial skin breaking out as it expresses our inner state of confusion. The skin is soft tissue, the mental energy, and a blemish therefore shows a mental irritation. This can result in emotional pain in the blemish itself. The skin will invariably clear as the inner turmoil or anguish clears. See also Acne, Chapter 6.

The Eyes

'The windows to the soul', the eyes are a deep expression of our inner being, the means through which so much can be read, understood, expressed and shared. It is here that contact is made and it is hard to hide our inner reality when this happens. If the eyes are vacant or distant we can see that no one is really at home, there is a sense of great emptiness within; if the eyes are full and bright, we can feel the inner joy emanating. All our different emotions are expressed through the eyes, from eroticism to distrust and hate. With our eyes we accept or reject, we caress or hurt. So completely do the eyes represent our whole being that there is a form of natural medicine associated with them: iridology. Through reading the lines and markings in the eyes an iridologist can infer what is taking place in the different organs and various parts of the physical body.

Not only do we communicate through the eyes, but we also see through them and thereby apprehend our reality. Vision problems are invariably connected to our interpretation of the world – such as not acknowledging inwardly what we are really seeing around us, and therefore not actually trusting our sight, or our inner vision. Near-sighted people tend to see only what is in front of them and have difficulty seeing beyond that to a greater picture. They also have difficulty projecting themselves and are often shy or introverted. It is as if the sight has been withdrawn or pulled back, maybe due to trauma or because of a fear of the future. Far-sighted people are happy seeing the great visions and vistas ahead, but have a hard time dealing with immediate, close-at-hand reality. They are the extroverts and adventurers, often out of touch with their inner feelings, or fearful of what the present may contain. Blurred vision can come about through not accepting reality as it is, when our inner reality does not mesh with the reality outside. Tension and stress also play an important role in determining sight, as such states easily distort our vision of how things really are. Poor eyesight may also be a reflection of how we see ourselves, as too humble or easily intimidated. To avoid confrontation of any kind we avert our eyes, or we develop bad eyesight and have to wear glasses. See Chapter 6 for more information on sight difficulties.

Our ability or not to accept what we are seeing will also be reflected in the health of our eyes. A client had contracted an infection that made her blind in her left eye by inflaming the optic nerve. She realised that at the time this happened she was not fully accepting the reality that her marriage was breaking up. The left side is our emotional, inner side. The eye becoming blind on that side showed her that she was blinding herself to her real emotions about the situation – emotions which indicated that her marriage was fast becoming intolerable. She was becoming inflamed and angry about what she was seeing. Through fully accepting the situation and allowing her real feelings about the relationship to be expressed, she was able to clear the infection.

Tears are a deep releasing of inner pain and hurt: being fluid they represent the outpouring and resolution of emotion. It is interesting to see how often one eye will be more closed than the other, or one will well up with tears while the other remains dry. The left eye represents the inner, emotional and intuitive aspect; the right eye is that which deals with the world and external situations, representing our more aggressive and assertive energies.

The eyes are connected to the Third Eye chakra, and thus the importance of the eyes in 'seeing', both physically and metaphysically. As we see outwards, so also we can see inwards, as in meditation when we turn the gaze inward and discover the inner world. Here lies the potential for transcendent wisdom.

The Ears

The ears are where we hear things; through them we take in our sound reality and then position ourselves according to that impression. When we are not happy with what we are hearing we will withdraw energy from that area or close off the hearing function. Often 'hard of hearing' is a very selective process. When talking with the elderly we soon find out how they can hear perfectly well when they want to, but immediately become hard of hearing when it is something they don't want to hear! I had one client who could easily hear me from across the room if I offered her a chocolate, but I had to shout for her to hear me if we started talking about her daughter, someone about whom she had nothing positive to say. Loss of hearing or earache can arise from being over-criticised, either by others or even by ourselves. In this case the daughter was all too fond of criticising her mother, and as a consequence her mother had stopped hearing her. Earaches can occur when what we are hearing is causing us pain and mental anguish, and is causing us to ache inside.

The ears are also our means of finding balance and therefore self-control and equilibrium. When our ears are out of balance it is invariably showing us that our lives are out of balance or out of control, that events are making us dizzy and uncentred. If we are not recognising what is happening in our lives then the ears will show us that we need to find a new balance and harmony. If only one side of our balance or hearing goes off, then we can look at the qualities inherent to that side (left or right, see Chapter 2) and apply them to what is happening in our daily reality.

The Nose

The primary use of the nose is to breathe: in combination with the lungs the nostrils take in air so that we may have life. This is not always a desired experience, especially on the unconscious level when things get bad and we want to stop what is happening. Consequently, at times when we are feeling particularly disappointed, disillusioned or powerless we may develop a bad cold with a blocking and closing down of the air passages, in an unconscious attempt to shut down the breathing or 'living' mechanism.

There is also another aspect that a cold represents, and that is the desire to cry, as will invariably be felt when we are feeling frustrated or hopeless. Many of the symptoms are the same, especially as both crying and a bad cold involve the release of emotions: the outpouring of fluid. So if we have a cold, we may want to ask if there is something we really want to be crying about. Is there a deep grief we are holding on to?

Although colds are infectious, it is worth noting who gets a cold and when. There are many millions of germs around us at all times, but there are only certain times when we become ill with one. Catching a cold is often synonymous with needing time out to reconnect with our inner selves and with our desire to live; it is a way of releasing pent-up frustration or emotions to do with inner change. Here we also find the sinuses, the passages of air that are connected to thought, to abstract realisation, awareness and communication. When they become blocked it is usually because we are mentally blocked, unable to communicate or go beyond our limited selves.

The nose is also our means of experience through smell. Particular odours can be associated with particular memories, and a blocking of the nose may be related to blocking off the memory of a painful situation. Smelling and breathing combined are the 'taking in of the smell of life', as when we smell a beautiful rose and experience joy in our whole being. As we develop in consciousness, so our nasal passages can become more sensitive to perceiving the metaphysical 'smell' around us.

The Mouth

The mouth is our direct means for communication. From here we express our feelings and thoughts, we take in food and nourishment and we begin the digestive process; here we kiss, smile, pout, snarl, spit, chew and bite. We take in our reality and throw it back out when it doesn't taste too good. Here too we speak, sing, whisper and shout.

With such a vast amount of uses, problems in the mouth are common. Difficulties can be related to having a hard time with tasting and then swallowing our reality; or a reluctance to digest what is going on; perhaps there is a lack of nourishment in our lives and therefore the mouth becomes starved. There may also be a desire to express negative thoughts and feelings that we think we should not express and therefore hold back in our mouths; or an inappropriate desire to kiss and love when we are actually being rejected.

The lips are particularly sensitive to our feelings. An example of this is Annie, who broke out in cold sores on her lips within two days of her honeymoon starting. Shortly after the cold sores began clearing up, she went into hospital with tonsillitis! The message was simple. The new marriage was bringing up many different issues that she did not want to deal with, so she expressed her confusion in such a way as to create a physical space around herself by stopping the kissing. At the same time she was finding it very hard to swallow what was happening: the reality of her situation was more than she had been prepared for. Unexpressed anger is particularly fond of finding an expression this way, and it can be anger with ourselves as much as with another person. Infections in the mouth indicate an irritation either with what we are taking in or with how we are expressing ourselves (See also Chapter 6.)

The Teeth

The teeth play a major role in the mouth as they represent the core energy or spiritual aspect, whereas the tongue and other soft tissue represent the mental aspect, and the saliva and other liquid the emotional energy. The teeth are like a gateway between ourselves and the outer world, acting as a filter determining what comes in and goes out. They deal with the first impressions of what we are going to be ingesting; incoming information, feelings and perceptions are separated here before they go on to be assimilated. Through chewing we break down our reality to have a look at it from the inside. In this way we can discriminate between what we want and what we don't want, spitting out what is unacceptable. If we clench our teeth it is like closing a gate, resisting what is coming towards us as much as holding back that which needs to come out.

Rotting teeth can indicate a breaking down of this discrimination process, an inability to assess and separate what is coming in from what we want to come in. This conflict can leave us quite vulnerable. It also means that what we are receiving is having an irritating, and therefore a rotting, effect on us. At the point of receiving there is a festering and reluctance, a pain in receiving. Rotten teeth in children can often be related to family problems and the conflict the child is having in what he is receiving. The guilt of these problems induces the parents to try to make up to the child by giving him or her sweets and chocolate, further stimulating the rotting process. The teeth are the first step in receiving love, nourishment and food; we depend on them to assimilate and to turn what we receive into a digestible form. If our teeth are useless then we are swallowing things that should not be swallowed – things that are painful to digest and integrate.

This was seen with Rosemary, who was having trouble with her teeth. She expressed that she was feeling irritated with her mother who was trying to get closer to her and dominate her life. Our mothers are intimately connected from infancy with love, food and nourishment, so this irritation was expressing itself in Rosemary's mouth, and in particular in her teeth that were trying to build a barrier against her mother attempting to get in. It was also indicating the need for her to actually express her feelings and talk with her mother, rather than clenching her teeth and holding on in the hope that her mother would just go away!

The teeth and the jaw are closely connected, for when we set or tighten our jaw we are also clenching our teeth. In this way we stop the swallowing and are able to hold on to everything exactly as it is without anything changing. We grind our teeth with anger; we pull back our jaw to stop ourselves expressing such anger, and this can accumulate so that the jaw muscles are actually pulled and distorted out of shape.

The Neck

In the neck we now come down from the abstract into physical conception, for it is here that we take in the breath and the food that will nourish us and give life to our physical existence. The neck is a two-way bridge between the body and the mind, allowing the abstract to find form and the form to find communication. Through the neck our thoughts, ideas and conceptions can manifest into action; at the same time our inner feelings, particularly those from the heart, can be released. Crossing this bridge at the neck demands a commitment to being here and to participating fully in life; a lack of commitment can result in a severe bodymind separation.

Through the throat we 'swallow' our reality. Difficulties in this area can therefore be associated with a resistance or reluctance to accept our reality and take it in. Food is what nourishes us and keeps us alive; it is a symbol of the nourishment in our world and is often used to replace such qualities. Yet how often were we told as children to 'eat our words', and thus to swallow our feelings? As Serge King writes in *Imagineering for Health*,

> We tend to associate food with ideas, as evidenced by such expressions as 'food for thought', 'do you expect me to swallow that?', 'you're feeding me a bunch of baloney', 'that idea is unpalatable', and 'he was force-fed with the wrong ideas'. The throat, then, and the glands and organs in and around it, can swell up and get sore as a repressed response to ideas that are unacceptable.

The same response will occur in connection to feelings from others or from situations that we are being asked to swallow, but that we find unpalatable.

Since the throat is a two-way bridge, problems in this area can equally represent the conflict in swallowing a reality that is unacceptable, as they can represent the frustration or repression of emotions trying to find expression, whether these be love, affection, pain or anger. If we believe that expressing these emotions is bad or wrong in some way, or if we fear the feelings or the consequences that such expression may have, then we will cut them off, causing the energy to amass in the throat. Such swallowing back of our feelings can result in tremendous tension in the neck and the associated glands. It is easy to see the connection of the neck with the fifth chakra as the centre of divine communication.

The neck also allows us the means to see on all sides, or to see all aspects of our world. When the neck becomes stiff and tense it limits our movement, thus limiting our vision. This indicates that we are becoming narrow in our views, narrow-minded, and are only open to seeing our own viewpoint, that which is directly in front of us. It also indicates ego-centred stubbornness or stiffness. Such stiffness limits the amount of feeling and communication we allow to pass between the mind and body. Cutting off or tightening in the neck clearly separates us from having to experience the responses and desires of our bodies, and from fully receiving input from our experience of the world around us.

Since the neck corresponds to conception, it also represents our feeling that we have a right to be here, that we belong, that this is our home. If that feeling is lacking, it can undermine our whole sense of security and presence, then a constriction or narrowing of the throat may occur. It then becomes very hard to swallow anything, thereby giving no energy or nourishment to our physical existence. It creates an 'opting out' syndrome, triggered through feeling rejected or hurt. This can also affect the functioning of the thyroid gland, as it is associated to the breathing mechanism and therefore to the taking in of the breath which gives us life.

The Shoulders

The shoulders represent the innermost aspect of our doing energy, that which expresses how we are feeling or thinking about what we are doing and how we are doing it; if we are doing what we really want to do or if we are reluctant in our activity; if we are being done unto or treated as we want to be. The shoulders represent the movement from conception down into matter and therefore action. Here we carry the weight and responsibility of the world, for now we are in physical form and have to confront all that being in form implies. The shoulders are also where the emotional heart energy finds expression as it moves up and out through the expressive energy of the arms and hands (through hugging and caressing). It is here that our innermost desires to create, express and execute are developed.

The closer we keep these feelings and conflicts to ourselves, the more tense and rigid our shoulders will be. How many of us are doing what we really want to do in our lives? Are we really free to express our love and caring? Are we hugging the person we want to be hugging? Do we want to participate fully in life, or would we rather hold back and stay locked away inside? Are we fearful to be ourselves, to act freely, to do what we want? To justify our holding back of such free expression we add further mental tension such as guilt and fear to our shoulders. The muscles then contort to accommodate these emotions. This can be seen in hunched shoulders, overburdened by the weight of life's problems, or the guilt from past actions; taut shoulders held high, rigid with fear and anxiety; or shoulders that are held back, thereby pushing the chest out as if trying to prove we can 'put up a big front' while the back is weak and distorted.

The muscles correspond to the mental energy, and it is common to find that energy knotted and gnarled in this shoulder area as it contains so many restrained desires. If the tension is predominantly on the left side, then it will be to do with the feminine aspect of our lives: maybe we are not fully expressing the feminine nature within us, or maybe the way we are handling the women in our lives is causing us concern. It also reflects the receptive and creative aspects, and our ability to express our inner feelings. Right-side tension is more to do with work and the masculine aspect, the expression of aggression or authority. This is the controlling and assertive side that takes on all of life's responsibilities. It will reflect our feelings about our activity in the world, as well as our relationships with men.

The shoulders are a means of expressing our attitudes, such as a shrugging of our shoulders to indicate we don't know what the right action is; a turning away from someone that shows we do not want to share ourselves with that person; or a moving of the shoulder forward as an invitation, often sexual. A cold shoulder can indicate that either we are receiving coldness from someone else, or we are giving it – our emotions are turning cold before we express them.

A broken shoulder indicates a much deeper level of conflict: a break in our deepest core energy as the tension between what we are planning or having to do, and what we really want to do, gets too much to bear. Recently a friend, Simon, was experiencing such serious communication problems with his wife that he had finally decided there was nothing else he could do but move out. It was Valentine's Day and he was shovelling snow off their porch when he took a step forward on to what he thought was the porch but proved to be just snow. He fell five feet to the ground below and badly broke the ball joint of his left shoulder. The implications of this break were enormous. Simon had made a decision to move out of the house, but his heart really did not want to; the conflicting energy between deciding to do one thing and wanting to do another was getting trapped in his shoulder. It was the left side, his emotional and inward side, expressing both his conflict with his own feelings as well as with his wife; and it was his bone, indicating that the conflict was an extremely deep one for him. The physical step forward that Simon took was an indication of the step forward he was planning to take, and it made him realise that it would actually be a step into the void. What he really wanted to be doing was paying more attention to what was in the house, and to the feelings deeper within him. As a result of the accident he was unable to move out as he became instantly dependent on his wife to do nearly everything for him.

This gave them both the opportunity to experience the more nurturing and caring aspects of their relationship that had become so fraught with negativity, and time to find a means for peaceful resolution.

The Arms

As the energy moves down the arms and into the hands it is going from the inward and personal aspects of our doing energy to the outward and more actively expressive aspects, as seen in our sense of achievement or competence. With these limbs we can either caress, hold, hug, give and reach out; or hit, take, push away; or fold up and protect our heart from anyone coming near. In this way the arms communicate and express our inner feelings and attitudes. This area is used as a means of communicating when we talk, as when we wave our arms to express much of what we are trying to say. The arms come outwards from our heart and are the extension of our inner being. Through them we also receive impressions and information about the world around us. Gracefulness or awkwardness here is a reflection of how we handle ourselves and our activities. A difficulty with assertiveness may be seen in the right arm, for this is the side that is predominantly to do with the masculine principle. A conflict with expressing gentleness and active love is more likely to be in the left arm, the side reflecting the feminine principle.

The Upper Arms

These parts of the arms are used to express strength and power. The tendency in men to over-develop these muscles often coincides with a resistance to expressing the heart energy, the softer, caressing and more caring aspects. It reflects a lack of grace and a desire to enter aggressively into activity, to become more 'masculine'. Conversely, under-developed or weak and thin upper arms can indicate a timidity in expression, a withdrawal from letting that energy flow forward. That withdrawal also indicates a weakness in entering into and actively participating in life, an inability to reach out and grasp hold of life.

The Elbows

Traditionally this is the place where we express our awkwardness as well as our pushiness, as indicated by the expression
'elbowing our way through'. We can just as easily elbow
someone out of the way as we can feel elbowed out; we stick our
elbows out to look brave and powerful, for they can enable our
arms to look like weapons. The elbows may also be expressing
doubt or conflict about our ability to respond or to be competent
enough to do something. The joints give freedom and gracefulness to our movement, and actually enable movement to take
place. If our elbows are locked, our ability to express ourselves in
many diverse ways becomes rigid, ungainly or even impossible:
try hugging someone with the elbows locked! Our elbows also
enable us to put effort into doing something, as with the phrase
'elbow grease'. If there is conflict in this area we may not be
asserting ourselves as much as we can do, or know we should be
doing.

The Forearms

These are an area of action, as when we roll up our sleeves to get
more involved in a situation. The forearms are also further away
from the inner expression and nearer to the outer expression of
our doing centre. The tenderness of the underside of the
forearms suggests the delicacy and hesitancy we may feel prior
to finally expressing something in the world, the moment when
it is still private yet about to become public; or when we are
doing something publicly, but only just below the surface we are
not entirely at ease about it.

The Wrists

Like the elbows, the wrists are joints that allow movement to
happen, for the doing energy to finally manifest outwardly. They
allow for tremendous ease and freedom to enter into our actions,
but when they are rigid our expression becomes jerky and clumsy.
In this way they make it possible for us to be flexible and accom-
modating in our handling of affairs, in the way we do things, in the
expression of our inner feelings. When the energy is freely moving

through our wrists then we are able to express ourselves freely: we are doing what we want to. When that energy is constricted (such as when we sprain our wrist or develop arthritis) it indicates a conflict in what we are doing; there is a rigidity permeating our actions; a restriction that hampers our activities; a pulling back from what we are doing; or maybe a blocking off from doing something that we know needs to be done.

The Hands

An intimate expression of ourselves in the world, the hands are like antennae going out ahead of us to feel the way and report back. When we extend our hand to another we are giving a message of friendliness and safety; a 'gentleman's handshake' is as good as the written word, for the power of touch goes beyond the rational mind. Here we paint, conduct music, write, drive, heal, chop wood, garden and so on. We become almost powerless if the hands are damaged, as it is through them that we normally interact with our world.

The whole of the gestation period is reflected here, particularly in the spinal reflex that runs along the side of the thumb. Our hands even have etched into them our entire past, present and future, and that which is unique to every human being: our fingerprints. I remember once when I was going through a period of intense personal and transformational work that the area of both my thumbprints became incredibly tender, almost raw. Both whorls began cracking and peeling, with all the old skin coming off like a snake shedding its outer layer. It was quite painful. I realised afterwards that it was as if I was creating a new person, a new 'identity', as I became free of past patterns and blocks. However, I never checked to see if my thumbprints had also changed!

Julie came to see me one day experiencing intense pain in her left thumb and left ankle. Her mother had recently died and the pain had begun shortly afterwards. When our parents die, it makes us realise we are no longer a child, we are now the 'end of the line'. Indirectly this makes us look at our own ability to be an adult, to become what we have lost, because we are now having to step into those shoes of 'adulthood'. Julie's pain had started in her left thumb as it related directly to the loss of her mother and the coming into adulthood that she was now experiencing in herself (the left side is the feminine principle). She was saying to herself, 'OK, I'm now the boss, I'm the next one up the line. I've moved up a generation.' The thumb was expressing the conflict in feeling that she had to be the boss, had to take control.

Then the pain spread to her ankle, the area which represents the support structure we stand on. The loss of her mother had undermined this support structure, one that Julie had relied on for so many years. As it was all on the left side it was directly confronting Julie with the doubts and fears of her own femininity, having just lost her most powerful feminine role model. Julie needed to see that it was not a matter of becoming the boss, or of stepping into her mother's shoes, but that she could find her own place and allow that to be different from her mother's. She began to acknowledge the conflict in herself because she had always wanted to go in her own direction and to do her own thing, but her mother had constantly disapproved of this desire in her. Now that her mother had died, Julie was feeling twice as much guilt in the idea of following her own direction.

The hands can easily become rigid and deformed through such afflictions as arthritis. A client I once saw had developed very painful arthritis in the fingers of her right hand, so that they were actually being pulled back out of shape. She told me she had been in a job for ten years that she really did not like, and now the arthritis had become so bad that she could hardly do the job anyway. She explained the arthritis as a feeling of being tightened and pulled back from the inside. This is exactly what her bodymind was doing. It was trying to show her that her resistance to her job was pulling her back, and the resistance was so severe that it was actually stopping her from working. A full acknowledgment of what she really wanted to do and a change of job quickly began to release this withheld energy.

As the fluids are associated with our emotions, so poor circulation resulting in cold hands indicates a withdrawal of emotional energy from what we are doing or are involved in; it can also mean a reluctance to reach out in an expression of love and caring. Conversely, sweaty hands indicate nervousness and anxiety, creating an excess of emotion, an emotional overflowing connected to our activity and involvement. The musculature of our hands is to do with our competence and ability to have a grasp on things. If we feel we are losing our grip, then the hands may reflect this through cramps, weakness or damage. Or they may reflect our feelings of incompetence, a fear of failing, of being unable to produce what is required of us. When we reach out too far, extend ourselves too much, or try to push ourselves forward at an inappropriate time, invariably we will cut, bruise, burn or otherwise damage our fingers.

Our hands are also our means of touching and connecting with another human being. The quality of that touching will say a great deal about us: it is a means of deep and silent communication. Touch is essential if we are to feel emotionally secure, confident, accepted and wanted; caressing, holding, hugging and stroking are vital ingredients for a healthy and balanced life. Without touch we become alienated and insecure, we feel rejected and unwanted; if seriously deprived of touch we can actually suffer mental damage. Through our touch we can help heal pain and suffering in another person. Conflict in our hands may indicate a great longing to touch or be touched in this way, but a fear of expressing this.

Being hesitant of touch indicates a deep fear of sharing ourselves, of exposing who we are, of allowing intimacy to develop. This may be due to previous abuse or because of natural introverted tendencies, but it is important to deal with this as prolonged reluctance will eventually cause more damage. Touch allows us to be open and vulnerable and therefore to be able to contact what is going on inside. Our hands enable that touch to take place. Hurting our hands may mean that we are resisting touch, trying to avoid such intimacy, as a way of avoiding confrontation with ourselves. It may also mean that we are being hurt through another person's touch – that the way they are handling or touching us is not acceptable and is creating pain.

The Back

The back is an interesting mixture of symbols and significance. On the one hand it is where we put everything that we have no desire to look at, or want to let anyone else look at; it is our dumping ground, the place where all the feelings and experiences that have caused us pain or confusion are buried. As we cannot see our back we become like ostriches, presuming that no one else can see either. Then we complain that we have a 'bad back', as if it had done something wrong! But on the other hand, apart from being our own personal garbage dump, the back also contains the spine, the most important part of our entire bodymind structure, the 'backbone' of our being, the underlying frame upon which the rest of our body is built.

The Spine

The series of bones representing the innermost core energy within us, and corresponding to our highest spiritual aspirations, our spine is the pillar upon which we rest; it is what makes us strong and competent, or leaves us appearing 'spineless'. It also connects with all the various aspects of our being through the skeleton, and through the central nervous system and the central blood supply running from the brain to the rest of the body. In this way every thought, feeling, event, response and impression is imprinted in the spine as well as in the relevant parts of the body involved. There are a number of different forms of medicine, such as Chiropractic, that focus on the spine, or the Metamorphic Technique, which focuses on the spinal reflexes. These systems recognise that through the spine we can reach and affect our entire being.

The spine is the first part of the physical body to be formed after conception; from here the rest of the body develops. It therefore represents our desire to incarnate, to come into being. Accessible through the spine is the pre-natal pattern, the development of consciousness during gestation (see Chapter 2). This pattern runs from conception at the neck to birth at the genitals; the movement here is one of growing maturity as the energy moves down the spine. But the spine also reflects the chakra system and the kundalini energy that starts at the base of the spine and moves upward. It can therefore be seen that our journey is one of leaving the infinite, coming in and developing as a human while the energy is moving downwards; and then moving back upwards through ever greater levels of awareness until we merge with the infinite again. Each part of the spine thus has two basic levels of energy operating within it: one is in the process of maturing as a human, and the other is the emerging of the Superhuman!

The Upper Back

By the upper back we mean the area from the shoulders down to the bottom of the shoulder blades. As this area reflects the post-conception time, or inward and personal development stage, so the issues that we dump here are invariably to do with feelings or confusions in relation to ourselves. This is the area where we are able to express our heart chakra and loving energy through our arms and hands. The aspect of this expression that is locked in the back is the love and warmth we feel for someone that we are unable to express and therefore hide, or the opposite of that, the anger or coldness that we do not want to admit. These feelings are trying to find a way out, but as they are continually ignored or denied they accumulate and can turn into repressed anger or rage.

Tight muscles creating an armour in the upper back are often loaded with rage that was initially aimed at ourselves but then gets projected outwards towards others. This can be seen in what is known as the 'dowager's hump', a formation of soft tissue that builds in the upper back, most often in older women. It would appear to represent a collection of angry and resentful thoughts that grow without the means for expression as the years pass; it manifests as we get older and as our reason or purpose for living loses impetus. (See also Chapter 6.)

Jim came to see me complaining of a relentless pain in his upper back. He had been to see numerous chiropractors, none of whom had been able to relieve this pain. He eventually began to tell me how, although he was divorced, his ex-wife would not leave him alone, was always phoning him, making demands, that she had literally become a 'pain in the back'. A few weeks after we started working together she upped and moved five hundred miles away, starting a new life of her own. Shortly afterwards Jim met a chiropractor who was able to fix his back in one session. Jim then realised it was because he no longer 'needed' the pain that it had been free to go, that he had actually been holding on to his ex-wife as much, if not more, than she had been holding on to him.

The upper back is also intimately connected to the shoulders and the energy that is expressed in that area, as described earlier. Pain or tension that manifests in this part of the back is therefore connected with frustration and irritation in not doing what we really want to do, with thwarted ambition or achievement. Invariably that is because we have cut ourselves off from our real inner desires and buried them in the back, perhaps because they were unacceptable or in conflict with what was expected of us. In releasing the hidden anger and frustration we can also uncover these long-hidden ambitions and aspirations. As this is the first stage of development after conception, it represents the coming into being, the manifesting of our inner purpose. This may mean simply finding our career or path in life but, on a higher level, it can mean leaving behind the lure and power of the material world in recognition of our spiritual intent.

The Middle Back

This is the area of our solar plexus, the small of our back, that so often seems to go out of balance. This area represents the quickening period, that time in the development of the foetus when there was a shift in consciousness from awareness of self to awareness of other than self. In other words, it is like the pivot on a see-saw that balances the inner, private aspects of our being with the outer, more public aspects. When this area is open and functioning then we are free to express our inner feelings outwardly and to give depth and meaning to our world. When it is closed or blocked it indicates a conflict in that expression, a holding back of the energy that should be freely flowing downwards, or a fear of expressing ourselves; it may be a reluctance to move our energy in an outward direction, for we feel safer when it is still inside.

As the movement downwards is one of growing maturity this is a natural blocking point, a holding back of the energy reflecting our inner resistance to growing older, responding to responsibilities or to facing our mortality. Here we are having to go from self to relationship, and this implies having to confront ourselves and deal with issues of adulthood and maturity.

This is also the area of the third chakra, that which is primarily to do with power and ego-identity. Disharmony in this part of the spine or back can therefore indicate power games or power conflicts, often activated in the process of discovering ourselves and our place in this world. The natural direction of our spiritual energy is to move upwards to experience ever higher states, but our ego will do everything it can to stop it! The lure and hidden promises of power are extremely seductive; once tasted, it is hard to say no to. However, this energy is closely related to corruption and manipulation. To rise above such seduction is the purpose of the spiritual path.

The Lower Back

This area runs from the solar plexus down to the coccyx, and it represents the final maturity before birth. Studies done on lower back pain have found that it is most likely to occur at those times that remind us that we are growing older; sixtieth and seventieth birthdays, wedding anniversaries, children graduating from college or leaving home, or retirement. Although gardening or lifting weights are usually labelled as the cause of back pain, it is more likely that there was already a weakness in that part of the back that then emerges through the excessive strain. The weakness is invariably this resistance to maturing and growing older within the context of society and relationships. In the West this is particularly prevalent as the emphasis is on being young, living longer and maintaining youthfulness as long as possible. There is little advice on how to grow old gracefully and with the dignity of mature wisdom. Lower back problems are also connected to the significance of the pelvis, as described below.

The Pelvis

This main area of the lower back merges with the energy of the spine, and represents relationship. Fears and conflicts to do with our security, our loved ones, family or friends are often found in this part of the back. The pelvis is the centre of movement within us, the area where we can give birth, not only physically but also to ourselves, as represented by the emergence of the kundalini energy, the coiled serpent of spiritual power, as it begins its journey upwards. As this energy begins to move, it needs expression. If we are incapable or fearful of such expression – for it can mean change and a deeper honesty in relationships – then we may close down in this area, causing stress, stiffness and pain.

The beginning of the journey upwards starts with self-survival, security and sexuality. Conflict with our sexual energy and expression is therefore found in this pelvic area, as is the fear of survival, or a fear of losing the ground we stand on. The pelvis is the pivot of the body, aligning the upward movement of the chest and head that is most exposed to the world, and the movement that goes out and down into the feet giving direction and grounding. It is from here that we go out to meet the world, and it is in here that we meet the reaction of the world to us. (See also Chapters 2 and 6.)

Jenny was sixty-five when we met. She had broken her hip three times in her life, always in the same place, and always because of an accident: the first time she fell off a horse, the second time was a car crash, and the third time she fell down a flight of stairs. The accidents were many years apart. After some talking and probing we uncovered the fact that Jenny had broken her hip for the first time two weeks after her fiancé had died, when she was twenty-one. She never married after this, but went to live with her parents and care for them. When she was forty-five, her mother died. A month later Jenny had a car crash and broke her hip again. When she was fifty-seven her father died. A few weeks later she fell down the stairs and broke her hip yet again. Each time she had broken her hip when the person on whom she was most emotionally dependent had died; when the security in her life was taken away. Each time she was given the opportunity to give birth to herself as an independent person, to learn how to stand on her own feet, she was unable to do it and the strain would weaken the hip so much that it would collapse. Jenny had to find herself as a separate person, she had to complete the maturing process, to find the security within herself in order to be able to walk forward easily again, free of depending on others.

The Buttocks

The lower back also encompasses the buttocks, the area we sit on and are therefore convinced that nobody can see. How many times have we had a smile on our face while our backside muscles have been clenched tight? As the buttocks are to do with elimination they are therefore connected to releasing and expressing feelings, emotions and sexuality. When they become tight and clenched it usually represents a real tightness in expression, a clamping down on being at ease. Try taking a deep breath and letting the buttock muscles relax, and feel the difference! Holding on tight here can cause strain and pain, distortion of the muscles and haemorrhoids. The anal muscles are intimately connected to childhood (such as potty training) and therefore with emotional conflict and repression; as well as with sexual conflicts (see discussion on the second chakra p.45).

The Chest

The area of the chest, from the neck to the diaphragm, reflects the post-conception stage which is the time of formation of the individual, the inner person. Therefore this whole area is to do with self in relation to self; it is our private and personal area (as opposed to the abdomen, which is to do with relationship to other). The Chest most directly symbolises 'I' and our sense of self-identity which we can see in the simple gesture of pointing to or touching our chest to indicate self, when we are talking about ourselves, our feelings or our opinions: remember Tarzan pounding his chest? This is where we 'put on a good front' to meet the world, puffing up with pride or self-assuredness, although we may be shaking with fear inside. This puffed-up chest is usually seen when we want to be in control and appear manly, when we can easily express our rage but have a hard time expressing our tenderness. If we have a contracted and small chest it can indicate that we are insecure and emotionally weak, timid in expression, needing security and reassurance from outside.

It is within the chest that we express many of our feelings, particularly to do with ourselves; these feelings may include our sense of self-value or self-dislike, our ability to love ourselves (from which we can then love others) and, conversely, feelings of anger or frustration with ourselves. Tension in this area will build a wall of armour, protecting against hurt or rejection. As Ken Dytchwald put it in *Bodymind*, 'The individual who holds tension in this bodymind region attempts to encase his heart and heartfelt emotions within a protective wall of armour. The armour guards against hurt and attack but also locks away feelings of warmth and nourishment.' It is this area of the body that harbours our innermost feelings which then find expression through our relationships, downwards through the pelvis and legs or upwards through the arms or the voice. Each of the organs in this area reflects a different aspect of this energy.

The Heart

Being made of soft tissue, the heart is a part of our mental energy, while its function is the distribution of emotional energy, blood. It is our symbol for love, on both the unconditional and the more personal levels. It represents all the romantic and lonely emotions that accompany love: we become broken-hearted, have heartache or leave our heart with someone or somewhere, depending on the circumstances. According to Serge King in *Imagineering for Health,*

> If compassionate you are 'bighearted', and if not you might have 'no heart' or be called 'hard-hearted' or 'cold-hearted'. A great loss might 'break your heart' and you may give 'heartfelt thanks' to someone else who is compassionate. In fear, your heart might skip a beat or find its way mysteriously into your mouth. All of these feelings have their biological reflections.

We express this heart energy through our mouth and lips, through our arms and hands, and through our genitals.

The heart is also connected to the heart chakra and therefore to the higher manifestations of love, namely the compassion and loving kindness that go beyond personal issues; but as this chest area of the body corresponds to post-conception, it is also to do with self. The message therefore is that we have to love and accept ourselves before we can really love others. True love is unconditional – it is love purely for the sake of love and not in order to get something in return; it has no limitations and is always constant. But we cannot develop this state if we are unable to feel it for ourselves first. If we do not love ourselves then there will be feelings of pain, inner anguish, self-dislike and denial underlying our attempts to love others; we will be loving others in order to be loved and feel better about ourselves. Our love is dependent on what we can get back in return, as we are unable to give to ourselves in the first place.

The heart is also associated with the thymus gland and therefore with the production of T-cells in the immune system. As described in Chapter 2, when we are experiencing positive and loving feelings our immune system tends to be stronger and better able to ward off infection. When the heart centre is not open but is experiencing negative emotions such as anger, hatred, frustration and self-dislike, then the thymus gland becomes weakened and the immune system reflects this in being less able to resist invasion.

Heart troubles are indications that this powerful centre of activity is out of balance, that there is a mental clamping down, a blocking or denial of experiencing love, or an inability to express it. There may also be a mistrust or deep fear of love – even the misbelief that we need to earn love through ruthless or materialistic measures. The typical heart attack comes at a time of financial pressure and competition, combined with a growing alienation from family and loved ones. Children are leaving home, years of hard work have denied time to be with them, the lures of younger women and shallow love affairs become easier to deal with than confronting the truth of the marriage, and so on. Heart problems are therefore telling us to slow down, take a look at what is important, and most of all to start loving ourselves and then to share that love with others. Denying this leads to a mechanical and dull life, or to stress that causes so much pain that the heart gives way under the pressure. Heart attacks are one of the top killers in the West, as we have become more and more isolated from our feelings, and from our involvement in and relationship to the natural rhythms of our world. Instead we have become obsessed with achievement and material gain.

In many traditional teachings the heart is seen as the centre of our being, even more important than the head, for it is from the heart that the warmth and love for all beings emanates. For instance, when we say, 'you have touched my heart', we are implying that the deepest level of our being has been affected. The American Indians were known to have said how strange it was to meet the white man, who 'thinks with his head instead of with his heart'. Endorsing this is the discovery of neurological links between the brain and the heart, indicating that the brain receives emotional input directly from the heart. As Alexander Lowen describes in his book *Bioenergetics,* the heart is like the king, with the mind acting as the king's advisers. The advisers go out into the world to see what is happening, then report to the king on the state of his kingdom, advising him on what to do. However, the king makes his own decisions based not on what each individual adviser might say, but on the overall picture. In this way the king may make a decision that can seem illogical to the advisers, but is actually the fair and correct one. In other words, if we are able to listen to our heart and make our decisions based on what it is saying, rather than on what the mind is saying, then we often find that the decision is the right one. It may not appear rational or logical; but if we follow it, then invariably it gives us greater happiness. In this way we can think with our heart.

As the heart is the centre of love and inner wisdom, so the blood takes that love and circulates it throughout our body; from loving ourselves we are then able to express that love and understanding throughout our world. The blood goes out and then returns to the heart; it gives and it receives. Blood also contains oxygen from the lungs; it is therefore the carrier of both love and life, that which permeates each cell of our being with purpose. Blood difficulties are a direct reflection of our relationship to this, invariably pointing to a sense of weakness, frustration or failure, an inability to cope or to respond; bad circulation indicates an inability to enter emotionally into the activity of life; constricted arteries imply a narrowing of our emotional movement, so that our expression and reception of love become restricted and limited. (See Chapter 6 for more details.)

The Lungs

When the lungs are being formed in the womb it marks our commitment to being here, to separate life, for this is what they represent. The taking in of breath is our saying 'yes' to life. The lungs can therefore also contain our fear of life, or a reluctance to being fully here. This gives rise to the tendency to want to be dominated by someone else: if we are not sure we really want to be here, it is much easier if someone else just makes all the decisions for us.

Breath is life, but we use only a small part of our full breathing potential. When we learn how to breathe fully and deeply we experience a new awakening of energy and enthusiasm for life. Shallow breathing is a way of cutting off such participation and feeling, a way of protecting ourselves from having to deal with relative reality. Anxiety and, fear, such as at times when our lives are being threatened, can trigger shallow breathing. Deep breathing puts us in touch with ourselves, with being grounded in our reality, enabling us to become fearless and at ease. Just as our lungs expand and contract, so they represent our ability to expand, share and enter into life, or to contract, isolate and retreat from life.

When we develop a cough or inflamed bronchial tissues we are often expressing an inner frustration or irritation with how we are feeling about ourselves. It may indicate that we have something we want to get off our chest, something we are trying to say or communicate that is blocked; there might be issues from deeper within that are coming to the surface, but we have not yet developed the courage or means to confront them. Or it may be that our personal lives and experiences are causing us irritation, making it hard to breathe in deeply. We do not want to take in, or to give out.

If we have asthma we may be manifesting a deep fear of separate life and the inability to expand into this separate life. We can be quite dependent, especially on one particular parent or a spouse. With asthma we are expressing a difficulty with being at ease in our world, such as having to live in a dust-free environment, as if earth was not really where we had meant to end up! There can also be a certain amount of guilt that we are not living up to expectations, or fear of rejection because we are not good enough. This indicates that we need to love and accept ourselves to the degree where we become free of needing another's validation and approval. (See also Chapter 6.)

Pam, an asthmatic client who was married and had a small baby, was visited by her mother for a week. Within ten hours of her mother leaving, Pam was in hospital having a severe asthmatic attack. On arriving at her own home two thousand miles away, her mother had to turn round and go back to her daughter's again. This time she stayed another two weeks before Pam was able to cope with her leaving. Pam had also had a severe attack on her wedding night, spending most of her honeymoon in hospital. When confronted with moments that clearly indicated that she had to stand on her own, the fear was too much to bear.

The Breasts

The principal symbol of femininity, the breasts provide joy, anguish, nourishment and comfort. They are the most over-exposed symbol of the whole body, with society proclaiming that they have to be a certain size and shape in order to be either fashionable or acceptable. Women agonise over their breasts, feeling insecure, inadequate and embarrassed. The left breast represents this on a deeply personal level, for the left side represents the feminine principle, the inner and more emotional aspects. The right side reflects the issues of femininity and being a woman in a largely masculine and aggressive world, the conflict between what is expected of us and what we are able or want to give; or how we see ourselves as women in the world.

The breasts are the providers of nourishment and life, both in the form of food and in the form of comfort and reassurance. However, if we are confused, unable or unwilling to express this life-giving quality, then it can turn into a rejection of our breasts and of the feminine nature that they represent. Breast cancer is intimately connected to our feelings about our femininity, our self-worth and our ability to express ourselves as women (see Chapter 6). It is equally connected to a fear of rejection by others, or a self-rejection.

Mary, for instance, developed breast cancer after having three children. She had been unable to deliver her children naturally (they were delivered through caesarean section) or to breastfeed them, even though she had desperately wanted to. She then became pregnant a fourth time, but miscarried. A year later cancer developed in her left breast. Mary was feeling an enormous amount of guilt and emotional pain, believing that she had failed as a woman, that she had not been able to be a proper mother. As she had been unable to breastfeed, the feelings of anger and rejection were directed towards her breasts. Her inability to carry a fourth child to full term added to her feelings of failure and hopelessness; her grief turned to anger towards herself. Her breast became the outlet of her emotions, as the symbol of her failure as a woman, and so it was here that she developed cancerous tissue.

Allowing the fullness of womanhood to emerge does not mean we have to have children, or have to be the best mother, or have the most perfect breasts. It means allowing the deeper qualities of womanhood to emerge – those of wisdom, intuition, love and compassion; the qualities of nourishment and caring. It is the acceptance and love for ourselves as we are, and the knowledge that the external manifestations are not as important as the inner qualities.

The Ribcage

The ribs form a protective cage around our most vulnerable and personal aspects: our heart and lungs. These organs give us separate and individual life, and the ribs are the guards that protect that life. When they break it is a signal that we are feeling unprotected, fragile or open to attack. We may have lost our sense of security, or be feeling as if we do not have any control over our own lives, and we are therefore helpless, exposed; we feel vulnerable at a deep core level.

The Diaphragm

A large flat muscle that separates the chest from the abdomen, the diaphragm acts like a gate between the upper part of our being and the lower. Through this gate pass the feelings and impressions from above that we must swallow down in order to assimilate and digest, and the urges and inspirations of the lower areas that need to move upwards to be expressed. Problems with the diaphragm, such as hiatus hernia, are an indication that this two-way flow of energy is in conflict. It may be a conflict with acknowledging our reality and allowing it to penetrate further into our being, or with feeling safe enough to express ourselves freely.

This area is also related to the quickening period, the time in the womb when the growing foetus begins to discover something other than self. It is the area of consciousness shifting from one state to another, of the inner becoming free to express outwardly and the outer expression finding meaning from within. If this area is blocked, then the inner energy becomes compacted and repressed, or the outer activity becomes shallow and empty, lacking depth.

The diaphragm is connected to our breathing, so a restriction in this muscular area means that we cannot breathe deeply – we are not wanting to take life into ourselves with fullness. It also relates to the change from the third to the fourth chakra, from lower to higher consciousness. As we move upwards from the solar plexus to the heart we are moving from a collective to a more individual level of consciousness, from selfishness to selflessness. The diaphragm has to be relaxed and open for this movement to take place.

The Abdomen

With the abdomen we now move into the area of relationship, for this is the pre-birth stage in the gestation period, where the foetus is preparing to move from a solitary state into a social one. Consequently any difficulties in this area are invariably to do with conflicts or blocks between ourselves and the world we are living in, expressed through the relationships that make up our reality. As this is also the area in which we can give birth to new aspects of our being, it is indicating how, through our relationships, through resolving conflicts that are inherent in those relationships, and by recognising our thoughts and feelings towards others and the world around us, we can grow and open to new areas within ourselves. This is the area where we take in, assimilate and 'digest' our reality, extract what is wanted and eliminate what is not wanted, where we hold on to or let go of personal issues.

What we have taken in from the outside gives us sustenance and energy; we can then use that energy to give back to the world. It is a continual process. However, if what we are taking in is causing imbalance, pain or indigestion, then we will not be receiving the nourishment we need and we will be depleted in energy. We will then have less to give back, and what we do have will be a reflection of the pain inside. This applies as much to thoughts, feelings, impressions and information as it does to food. Our abdomen is where we process our reality, then build ourselves upon that reality, and finally share the result with others. If our reality is painful and abusive then we are more likely to give pain and abuse in return. If it is warm and loving, then we will be well nourished and our own loving and creative energies will be free to express themselves.

This area is closely connected to our inner thoughts and feelings, recognised in such statements as 'having a gut feeling', 'having no guts', or being 'unable to stomach it'. Here resides our deepest intuition and sense of what is right or wrong; a response in our stomach is often a better guideline to what is going on than our sensory impressions may be. When we have a strong gut feeling we can guarantee it will be right; to ignore it will often lead to a bad feeling inside and mistakes made outside.

The Stomach

Food represents mother, love, affection, security, survival and reward. We replace our need or desire for any one of these with food as a way of filling the emptiness within. We use food instead of affection and love, especially at times of loss, separation or death. We also use it to ease financial or material tensions. Eating sweet food is a way of feeding ourselves the sweetness we crave, of temporarily giving to ourselves the sweetness or reward that we may feel nobody else is giving us. Conversely, in expressing our need for nourishment we may also stop eating, thereby reducing or shrinking our need for affection to a level that makes no demands at all. In this way obesity and anorexia are actually expressing a similar state: that of not loving self and therefore needing outside reinforcement and affirmation, but not receiving that affirmation enough to satisfy the demand. The reaction to that state is simply expressed in opposing ways: obesity indicates a loss of personal control, while anorexia implies a highly exaggerated attempt at control. (See Chapter 6 for more information on these conditions.)

All this is dealt with in the stomach. Here the longings, unfulfilled desires, worldly pressures and external conflicts are first assimilated. Little wonder that they can cause so much upset, such as indigestion, ulcers or acidity. How often do we hear someone say that something is 'eating away' at him, and then we also find that he has a stomach ulcer? The stomach modifies and breaks down the food and renders it capable of being absorbed, before sending it further down. Food can spend many hours passing through the stomach, so it is not surprising to find that thoughts and feelings can also sit in here for a long time, creating nausea and tension. A rigidly tense stomach area can indicate a resistance to allowing issues to pass through, a holding on to reality in an attempt to prevent inevitable moves and changes.

The Intestines

From the stomach the food passes down into the small intestine and then into the large intestine, or colon, before elimination. In the intestines we absorb the nourishment and separate the good from the bad. This involves a process of integration and letting go, not just of food but also of feelings, thoughts and experiences. If this process of letting go is restricted (due to insecurity, fear and so on), then a holding on takes place and constipation, intestinal ulcers or a spastic colon can develop. If the letting go is too hasty and thereby reduces the integration time, then diarrhoea can follow.

The intestines are where we hold on to those issues we are fearful to let go of, where our outer reality connects with our inner reality, and where we eliminate that which we no longer want to have inside us. As Bernie Siegel explains in *Love, Medicine and Miracles*,

> After emergency surgery to remove several feet of dead intestine, a Jungian therapist recently told me, 'I'm glad you're my surgeon. I've been undergoing teaching analysis. I couldn't handle all the shit that was coming up, or digest the crap in my life.' Any connection with her feelings might not have occurred to another physician, but it was no coincidence to us that the intestines were the focal point of her illness.

In 1982 I was travelling through Egypt. I arrived in Cairo late at night and was driven from the airport through the city to the hotel. I felt like I was being emotionally hit in the guts. It was even more emotionally disturbing than when visiting Bombay or Delhi because in Egypt, in July, it is so very hot and dry that there is no green foliage or water anywhere; at least in India there were trees and flowers. But here there were more than 12 million people living in a dry and dusty city built for 3 million. They were living in every place imaginable, including the graveyards. Within a few hours of arriving I was emptying my intestines at a rapid rate! I had become infected with a parasite of some sort, but the reason it happened then, and with such force, was because my intestines were already emotionally weakened and in pain. I had literally been hit in the guts by what I was experiencing.

A few years later I had a recurrence of the parasites while I was working in the psychiatric ward of a nursing home. The level of suffering around me was so great that I literally took it in my guts as I had done earlier in Egypt. I then realised that the parasites were actually living off the suffering that I was absorbing. My healing meant that I had to learn how to be objective and free from taking on the suffering; how to be compassionate and unconditionally loving yet without getting subjectively involved in the reality I was witnessing.

Constipation is a holding on, a tightening of the muscles so that elimination, or release, cannot take place. The constipated personality arises when we are controlling and dominating and have a hard time being spontaneous. This can be due to a fear of events getting out of control, as much as a fear of expressing our creative nature. Allowing life to unfold in its own way is one means of dealing with this. But it is not always easy: the very nature of constipation is to hold on, and this holding on will be as much to the illness as it is to the emotional causes of that illness! We spend a fortune each year on laxatives, for fear is a common human condition, especially fear of loss, or insecurity. We are much more likely to have constipation when we are experiencing financial problems or relationship conflicts, or when we are travelling. These are times when we are feeling insecure and ungrounded; we want to hold on to everything as it is and not let it change, as we do not know what will come next. However, in so doing we create deep tension as well as pain and irritation. Letting go means trusting that it is safe to let go, trusting that life will resolve itself and that we do not have to have the power in our hands in order for the world to function. It means learning how to play, how to express ourselves freely, and how to be at peace with whatever happens.

There are those times when the reality we are having to digest is upsetting, overwhelming or fear-provoking, and we have no desire to hold on to anything, let alone absorb any information from the situation. Then we tend to have diarrhoea, just like an animal that empties its bowels when confronted with a life-threatening situation. However, we are most prone to suffer from recurring diarrhoea if we are the type that rushes through things without stopping to listen and absorb what is being said. We will therefore lack nourishment and fortitude, as there are no reserves to fall back on. Here the message is to slow down, take time to listen and absorb one situation fully before moving on to the next.

The Liver

This organ is literally that which gives and maintains our lives. All the blood from the stomach and the intestines passes through the liver, allowing for full and proper absorption of nutrients. The liver absorbs and stores fats and proteins, as well as helping to maintain the sugar level in the blood. It is essential in detoxicating poisons that enter through our digestive system, and therefore plays an important role in the immune system. The liver can even regenerate its own tissue.

As the liver has the function of absorbing nutrients from the blood, it can also be said that it plays the same role with our emotions. In traditional Chinese acupuncture the liver is known to be associated with anger, so here we can see how the liver absorbs the anger out of our blood, thus keeping us in a balanced emotional state. If it did not perform this function we would soon become emotionally overwrought or repressed. However, the liver is also a storehouse for nutrients and in the same way it is known to store anger, to be a place where anger can be deposited and even cause damage if not recognised and released. Anger towards ourselves can lead to depression; as depression grows, it can cause a sluggish or malfunctioning liver.

The liver detoxicates bodily poisons and in so doing helps keep us sweet and healthy. But it can also become a repository for those poisonous aspects of our being, for the bitter and resentful thoughts and feelings we may have but are not expressing or resolving. The liver's role in the immune system emphasises how influential negative thoughts and feelings can be in relation to our general state of health. As the anger or bitterness accumulates, so the liver will feel the strain and not be able to function fully. This will then affect not just the liver but also the blood and immune systems, and therefore our ability to fight infection.

The functioning of the liver is very involved in addiction behaviour, whether the addiction be to food, alcohol or drugs, as it is the liver that removes the toxins from the blood and deals with the excess fat and sugar intake. The emotional tension that gives rise to the need for release through an addiction is felt here, as this tension may be based on anger and resentment (towards the world, or towards specific individuals). Often the toxins are ingested through the addiction as a way of hiding from those toxins already in our own system: hate, frustration, rage, incompetence, self-dislike, hurt, greed and a need for power. By taking in external toxins we do not have to admit to, or face up to, what is already inside us.

The liver is closely connected to the third chakra, that which focuses on power and self-identity. By transforming these qualities we are able to rise above them to the higher levels. But it can be just as easy to become a victim of these energies as it can be difficult to transform them. The liver then reflects the anger and confusion experienced in trying to find ourselves and our purpose.

The Gall Bladder

This small organ has a descriptive language that tells us clearly what is going on. The function of the gall bladder is to enable fats to break down through the use of bile, made in the gall bladder. 'Gall' is usually associated with guts or courage, but also to irritation and insensitivity. 'Bile' is associated with bitterness, with something feeling very sour or bitter inside. Lack of bile means that fats do not get properly digested and we feel queasy and upset. So problems in the gall bladder can be associated with mental and emotional patterns of irritation and bitterness towards other people, or with situations in our lives that upset us. These thought patterns can congeal and harden, becoming gallstones that may be very painful to release. The power of negative thought is not to be underestimated!

The Pancreas and the Spleen

Although these two organs have their own individual functions they are both involved in the secretion and distribution of insulin. The pancreas maintains the sugar balance in our blood; without it the sugar level rises and causes innumerable problems such as diabetes. Hypoglycaemia is the opposite of this, where there is not enough sugar in the blood, and weakness and dizziness can occur.

The sugar level in our blood obviously relates to the amount of sweetness and love in our lives and to the opposite, anger and sourness. Diabetes can indicate that the love we are receiving is uncontrollable and excessive, to the point where it is smothering or overwhelming. It is also unusable as it is constantly being eliminated in the urine, thus responding to a sense of loss and inner sadness. In this state there is a great desire for affection and love, yet an inability to know how to act if it is received. This gives rise to anger and resentment, a blaming of others for our own inner fear and confusion in dealing with love. The word spleen also means moroseness and irritability. Hypoglycaemia indicates the same conflicts with expressing and receiving sweetness, but the conflict leaves an inner depletion and emptiness. (See also Chapter 6.)

The Kidneys and the Bladder

The process of waste disposal, of cleansing the blood of harmful waste products while maintaining its nutrient balance, is begun by the kidneys. The bladder is the collecting chamber for the waste fluid before it is released. This part of our bodily system is intimately concerned with the cleansing and release of negative emotions (urine). As this is the area of the pelvis, remember that these emotions are primarily to do with self and other, with relationship, with our reaction and interaction with the world around us.

The kidneys are connected to the adrenal glands (one gland sits atop each kidney) and to adrenalin, which is released at critical and stressful moments when the 'flight or fight' syndrome is activated. In other words, the kidneys are associated with fear: fear of relationship, fear of expression (especially expressing negativity), and fear of self-survival. Whether to 'fight' and go outside for answers and release, or whether to 'flight' and go inside for resolution, becomes an issue here. Kidney stones usually develop through dehydration when the urine becomes crystallised; this can occur when we are holding on to old thoughts or attitudes that should have been released, or past sadness (tears) now taking form. The release creates the opportunity for movement into a whole new free state of being, as we let go of the past.

The kidneys are connected to the third chakra, as seen in Chapter 3, and also to the second chakra, sexuality and sexual issues (and therefore relationship issues), as is the bladder. Here the emphasis is on adaptability, as the bladder has the wonderful ability to adapt to varying amounts of urine (negative emotion) passing through it. In *Traditional Acupuncture: The Law of the Five Elements* Dianne M. Connelly writes:

> Adaptability is a key characteristic of the functioning of the bladder and this is significant on every level. A person prone to deep depression, inability to cope with life situations, or fears of change, may have an energy imbalance in which the key problem is the inability to adapt. Being able to urinate is a part of the process of flow within the entire bodymindspirit.

This is clearly demonstrated in research showing that cases of cystitis (inflamed bladder) are more common during and after the break-up of a relationship. During this time there are invariably many negative emotions that are not being voiced: hurt pride, anger, fear of being alone, loss and rejection, and sexual inadequacies – to name but a few. These unexpressed emotions begin to accumulate and cause intense irritation and frustration. Cystitis is an irritation of the urinary system, the system that is our means to release the emotions we no longer need and that cause damage if retained. As this is in the area of the pelvis, so it is emotional energy to do with relationships. During a relationship separation the emphasis is also on having to find ourselves anew, having to stand on our own feet rather than being dependent on another person. This is the symbol of the pelvis, the area where we can give birth to ourselves. The cystitis is telling us that there is a build-up of negative emotions that need to be released, alongside the need for us to begin now to find our own independent ground to stand on.

The Reproductive Organs

The whole of the reproductive organs are naturally connected to sexuality, to our innermost feelings about our femininity or masculinity, our acceptance or rejection. Here is our ability to create new life, and in so doing to share of ourselves with another through sex and procreation. Problems in this area are a manifestation of inner conflicts and confusions, difficulties in communication, in sharing, in being at peace with ourselves and with the opposite gender, in being free and able to trust, in being respectful and considerate. Sexual problems such as impotence or frigidity highlight deeper issues of past pain, trauma and abuse, insecurity, feelings of inadequacy and failure, self-dislike, guilt and neglect.

Sexual energy is one of the most powerful expressions in the whole bodymind, for it is the energy that resides at the base of our journey downwards into birth and maturity, and at the beginning of our journey upwards through the chakras to the higher states of awareness. Through this energy we can dissolve the ego, give birth to new understandings and inner freedoms. It is a place of tremendous transformation. In tantric yoga the power of the sexual energy is used to awaken the kundalini, the coiled serpent that rises up the spine through the chakras. In this practice there is no ejaculation, for the energy of the orgasm is used to go up rather than out. This practice is just one example of how very important our sexual energy is. It is an energy that enables two people to unite and merge, thereby releasing their egos and attaining a true oneness. It is a way of expressing our deepest feelings of love and care for another. It is also a means to work with and resolve conflicts that are holding us back from true growth.

However, throughout the ages sexual energy has been misused and abused, particularly when its higher potential is ignored in favour of purely sensual indulgence without real feeling, for exertion and manipulation of power, and perversion. When the deeper purpose and beauty of sexual energy is denied in this way it can turn inwards on us and implode, as it has no means of finding true fulfilment in expression. It will then create different problems such as sexually transmitted diseases: literally a dis-ease, or unease, within the sexual energy.

The Legs

Extending from our moving centre, the pelvis, the legs take the moving energy outwards into the world and represent our direction and motion. With our legs we are able to walk and run, to find rhythm and purpose to our movement. Through them we are grounded – we recognise and relate to the earth as the body or place from which we have evolved – from this place we can then draw support and stability, much as a tree draws support from its roots in the ground. The energy flows upward from the earth giving us a sense of firmness, of being strong and well rooted. It also flows downward from the body into the earth, releasing energy and keeping us in touch with reality. Our legs express this level of groundedness or firmness, as well as the passage of life we have experienced and the direction we are now going in.

The legs also represent our standing in the world, and therefore how others see us. They communicate our ability to 'stand on our own' or not. Standing on our own legs and feet obviously marks our independence, as well as our difference from other animal forms. Weak legs tend to indicate the lack of this energy passing through them, the lack of groundedness, or an inability to stand up for ourselves and be strong in our own world. There will be a tendency to be dependent on others; as our own movement is weak and uncertain, we look to others for motivation and support. The opposite of this is very well-developed legs, with big muscles. Here the energy is so rooted in the ground that there is little room for spontaneity or change in direction. There is likely to be a tendency for repetition, to always be following the same path or direction, even if there is little enjoyment. There may also be a fear of reaching out and opening up emotionally. Fat legs are similar to this, only less conscious. Here there is more apathy and a lack of response; a wall of mental patterns stand between our inner motivation and our ability to put that motivation into action. Conversely, tight, lean legs are full of energy but the energy is not flowing gracefully – it is raring to go but has not found a means of expressing itself smoothly and peacefully. It can then become brittle, breaking or collapsing at the joints.

Tight muscles and tension in the legs are to do with our relationship to the ground. There may be conflict with the direction we are taking, or a sense of insecurity as if the rug could be pulled from beneath us at any moment. This latter issue is fairly common when an insecure childhood, or other similar trauma, has been experienced. Then there is a built-in fear and uncertainty, a reluctance to trust the ground as being solid or able to support us. Tension in the leg muscles results from a holding on for fear that if we let go we will fall or be 'let down' in some way. Muscle tension can also result from a reluctance, or 'holding back', from where we are going. If there is doubt or resistance to the direction and movement that is happening in our lives, then the legs will try to hold back that movement.

The Thighs

Being nearest to the pelvis, the thighs tend to represent the more inner and personal aspect of moving. Issues here can be closely associated to sexuality, to expression, to being able to share ourselves and our movement with another. This is intimately connected to our sense of femininity or masculinity. Issues to do with our parents are also found here, as we have to move away from the parental energy (in the birth area/pelvis) as we grow and mature. Excess weight in this area is like a build-up of mental resistance to fully expressing or finding our own direction, and to being at peace with our sexual expression; it is a way of blocking off from really experiencing the depth of our feelings in this part of our bodymind.

The Knees

To find out what the knees represent, try walking with locked knees and see how it feels! Immediately there is a rigidity, a stiffness and inflexibility. So the knees represent the ability to bend, to be giving and to be spontaneous. The knees are where we kneel, an act associated with surrender or acknowledgment of higher authority. They are where we express our pride and humility. A difficulty with the knees can be a difficulty with giving in – with accepting the situation and surrendering to it – due to our arrogance or stubbornness. They give us flexibility and are our shock absorbers, absorbing the pressure from above and from the ground below that we are walking on.

In T'ai Chi Chuan, the Chinese form of moving meditation, the knees are kept bent throughout the practice. This releases the flow of energy, as locked knees will keep the energy locked and unable to move freely. The same posture is used in Bioenergetics, enabling the energy to flow through to the ground. Joints allow us to be either fluid and to move gracefully, or they lock us up and produce jerky, 'disjointed' movement. They are gathering points for energy and can easily become blocked and tense. When there is resistance to movement or change, a reluctance or stubbornness to surrender, too much pride, or a fear of progress, then the knees will feel the strain.

I remember many years ago when I was the manager of a vegetarian restaurant and new owners bought the business. They had never done anything like this before, so as manager I offered to help them and show them what I knew. However, they wanted to learn for themselves and I slowly watched them make one mistake after another. It was hard for me to accept the situation and I kept trying to teach them how to do it; then my pride would get hurt when they took little notice of what I said! During this time my knees began to get very painful, and I could hardly get up in the mornings due to the aching stiffness. The day after I finally accepted that it was time I resigned was the day the pain in my knees went away. I had surrendered!

The Shins

This part of the legs is closer to the feet and to the more worldly and external expressions of our movement and direction. The lower leg represents the energy of this movement just prior to manifestation, before activity has happened but when it is definitely pending. For instance, a friend of mine was in the middle of reluctantly packing her belongings to move to another town. It was not really what she wanted – she would have preferred to stay in the house and place she was in – but she had little choice. In the process of packing, she kept tripping over objects on the floor, badly bruising her lower legs. Her mental resistance to the move was showing itself, even though the move had not yet happened.

The Ankles

Like the knees, the ankles are joints that have an immediate relationship with the direction we are going in and our ability to cope with that direction. However, the ankles have an added symbolism for they are the bridge between the body and the feet, between above and below, between the mind and the earth. In this way, if energy is not flowing smoothly into the ground it may get built up here. The achilles tendons bring the mental and bodily thoughts and desires into realisation, as well as expressing any blocks in this movement. For instance, we might have a strong desire to get settled, to find or put down roots, to discover a place in this world for ourselves. But at the same time it may be impossible to manifest this quality, perhaps due to a job that keeps us on the move, or not enough money being available. When this happens, a block will develop between the desire for the energy to move downwards to the earth, and the available receptivity in the feet. The ankles express this blocked energy.

The ankles also represent our mental and spiritual support structure, the set of values and concepts that we stand on. They represent who we are in the world. When the ankle gives way, our whole body collapses. If the ankle is twisted or sprained it represents a twisting of this support structure – nothing is clear and straightforward any more, but is confused and distorted. The direction we are going in and the events that that direction is determining are in conflict with our inner support structure, or may be giving rise to fear and confusion. The unconscious desire is to change direction, to straighten out the twists in our lives. This can happen at a time of trauma or unexpected change, when we get confused about where we should be going. A broken ankle bone represents this conflict on a much deeper level, a very deep hurt or confusion about our standing, security, purpose or direction in the world. Twists, sprains or breaks halt our movement forward for a period, during which time adjustments and an acceptance of the situation can be made.

The Feet

An extraordinary part of the bodymind, the feet actually have reflected in them the maps of many different aspects of our being. One of these maps, such as that used in Reflexology, is a guideline for treating the body on a physical level, for the feet reflect the body and all its internal organs. Another map, the one used in the Metamorphic Technique, is that of the time period from conception to birth. (See Chapter 2.) Through our feet we can therefore be in touch with both our physical and our metaphysical being.

Here we are also in contact with the earth, and in this way the feet communicate our whole being to the world. They are that part of us that moves forward first and furthest, that extends itself outwards. They represent our passage on earth. If we walk with both feet turned outwards, then there may be some confusion about where we are going; if our feet are turned inwards, then it can be saying that we are unclear in our direction. The feet are the platforms we stand on, our grounding and balancing points, as well as the instigators of our movement. Imbalance here throws the whole of the rest of our being off balance.

The physical state of the feet can indicate much of what is happening in our lives. The toes represent the head and all the different sensory functions that take place there. The big toe is particularly interesting as it has reflected in it the pineal and the pituitary glands, the crown and the Third Eye chakras. This area represents the more abstract and spiritual part of us. Ingrown toenails, which usually occur on the big toe, therefore represent a conflict between the mental (soft tissue) and the spiritual (hard tissue) energies in this thinking and creative area. I remember experiencing this at one point when I was writing *The Metamorphic Technique*. At the time I felt as if my head was in an iron cage and I could not reach beyond it to greater wisdoms or insights. As I finally broke through the mental barriers that were stopping my creative flow and I was able to reconnect with my spiritual understanding, so the toenail condition improved!

Hammer or withdrawn toes indicate stress and reluctance to moving forward, as well as resistance to or fear of an abstract and more unstructured way of being. Clutching toes express a desire to run away, to find another means to move forward, or another direction. The neck and the conception point are just below the joint of the big toe, and if we follow on down the side of the foot, which is the spinal reflex area, so we move through the different areas of the gestation period until we reach birth at the heel. (See Chapter 2, Fig. 2.) The balls of the feet are the chest area, the arch is the solar plexus area, and the underside of the heel is the whole of the abdominal organs.

A bunion develops on the foot at the point of the post-conception stage shortly after conception, at the time when in the gestation period the lungs are being formed. The lungs represent our separate self-support system. The bunion can thus indicate a weakness, almost a reluctance, in our decision to stay here and continue with individual existence at this time. This manifests later in life in the form of immaturity and a need for a dominant relationship: due to our not really wanting to be here, it is much easier to have someone else make all the decisions for us. Bunions usually arise at the time of entering into such a dominant relationship, whether it be with our parents, with a dominating mate or even with our own children. Owning ourselves and our place in the world, taking responsibility for ourselves and thus entering more fully into being here, can enable a bunion to change.

As the arch corresponds to the solar plexus area and therefore to the quickening period, so it can be seen as representing the movement from awareness of self to awareness of other than self, or from private to public. Flat feet therefore indicate that we have no boundaries, no separation between inner and outer, leaving us very vulnerable and unprotected. There are no boundaries, yet we need boundaries in order to define ourselves. To avoid confronting this vulnerability, if we are flat-footed, we will skim over the surface of things, never fully entering into them, never completely putting down roots, always on the move. Seeing no separation between work and private life, the two often overlap, invariably to the detriment of the rest of our relationships. This also makes for a more shallow and unimaginative way of being. Conversely, if we have high arches then we have drawn a very clear line between private and public, rarely allowing the two to overlap. Because of this we can seem quite aloof and withdrawn, intensely private; not often will we make the first overtures towards friendship. High arches can indicate intense creativity, like the withdrawn artist producing masterpieces that few other people ever get to see.

The heel represents mother earth, a sense of coming into reality. If we walk around on our toes it can feel as if we are avoiding reality, pretending we are not really here as our head is in the sky and there is no contact with earth. As we bring our heels down there is a corresponding connection with the ground and the world. If we dig our heels into the ground we are showing a desperate attempt to be grounded, to hold on to reality at all costs, probably because of a deep insecurity that it will be taken away. A build-up of dead or peeling skin indicates a build-up of mental patterns and thoughts no longer needed but not yet let go of. This is the area of birth, therefore of being able to give rise to newness and to manifest potential.

Swollen feet are to do with our emotional state, a holding of emotional energy to do with the direction we are going in. Sweating feet are a release of this emotional energy, indicating an excess of emotion. Blisters occur at times of friction in life, when mental and emotional issues are causing conflict or rubbing us the wrong way. We think that it is a shoe that is causing the problem, but in fact the weakness was already there and the shoe is simply a catalyst. In the words of Robert St John in *Metamorphosis*,

> Normality of function is without stress. Normal tissue [tissue that has no disturbance] has a positive response to the pressures and irritations imposed upon it. A normal foot will fit into an unsuitable shoe without resistance in just the same way that a normal person will fit into different elements of society without friction.

Having completed our journey through the body in this way, we can now look at all the different aspects of dis-ease or disorder with our new bodymind understanding.

CHAPTER 6

From Abscesses to Ulcers

There are no incurable diseases, only incurable people.
                    DR BERNIE SIEGEL

THIS chapter is by no means a definitive list of ailments, diseases or difficulties, merely an easy-reference, alphabetical guide to the most common ones. If a particular ailment is not listed here, start by going through the previous chapters to bring all the different patterns together. It is important to recall that the inner correspondences of most problems can usually be traced to within the six to twelve months before the onset of the problem. Occasionally we need to go back further than that, or we find related incidents from recent times that connect to the present state.

Let us remember that the body will be manifesting the *unconscious* patterns, not the conscious ones, for it is the unconscious energies that are trying to make themselves known to us. These are the attitudes and patterns that we are not recognising or acknowledging in the conscious mind. The descriptions mentioned here are simply to help us delve deeper into the unconscious and therefore to come to know ourselves more fully, to see what it is in ourselves that we are not looking at. Healing, or becoming ease-full, will be discussed in the following chapters, unless immediate guidelines are appropriate here.

Abscess: A collection of pus that either erupts by itself or has to be cut open. An abscess indicates an angry or hurt emotional response (pus is fluid/emotion) or feeling that is fermenting, becoming irritated and inflamed; finally it has an effect on the mental energy as well, producing mental upheaval (swelling). The eruption leaves us empty and exhausted. The particular emotion will be associated with the function and the part of the body where the abscess appears. For instance, if it is in the leg it will be connected to the direction our lives are going in and resistances or conflicts about that direction; or with our ability to stand up for ourselves, to express our independence and freedom. *See also entries on the side and part of the body affected.*

Accidents: This indicates a need for direct and immediate action as the mind is using an extreme situation to express itself, often involving an actual stopping of the direction we are going in. The conflict may have been unfolding over the previous year, as the part of the body damaged through the accident is usually already in a weakened state; the accident brings that weakness to the surface for us to see. The unconscious need for change, for complete reassessment, is so great that it is dramatic. *See also entries on the side and part of the body damaged, and on the nature of the damage.*

Accident-prone: This situation arises through a conflicting relationship to reality, an inability to being fully present and aware of the world as it is presenting itself; we may instead want to be elsewhere. We are ungrounded in what is happening around us, maybe because our reality is unacceptable or difficult to relate to. We need to become more grounded and to discover our security and inner trust.

Ache: When felt in the muscle, this sort of pain indicates a mental ache, a mental longing, a desire for something that is not being fulfilled. This is energy being blocked in the muscle when it should be passing through and being expressed, so it indicates an ache for activity and movement, for change and fulfilment. Ache in the bone is a longing that affects us on the deeper, inner levels, an ache in the very core of our being. A deep pain and longing is being expressed. *See also entries on the side and part of the body and tissue structure affected.*

Acne: The face is where we face the world, that part of us seen first, and where we are accepted or rejected. When we are in conflict emotionally and mentally with who we are, with expressing our inner nature, with discovering ourselves, then conflict can erupt. Acne is an expression of anger, resentment and fear, all connected to finding and establishing our own self-identity, to being unconditionally accepted and loved for who we are as an individual. Sadly, acne often makes this self-discovery even harder, as it can create inhibition and embarrassment. It is known that junk food can cause acne: it affects the functioning of the liver, which is our storehouse for anger (*see Liver and p.87*). Acne can be a way of avoiding contact with others, that even though we may long for such contact, we are fearful of it. Acne also indicates we are being picked on, allowing something to get under our skin and create negativity. *See also Face and p.57.*

Addictions: An addiction is the attempt to find fulfilment in something outside of ourselves, as the ability to fill that need from within is lacking. Addiction may be to food, cigarettes, drugs, alcohol, sex and so on. Whatever it might be, it is a means of filling the emptiness, the hopelessness, the meaning-lessness of life that is like a deep hole inside, demanding satisfaction. This is an issue of our relationship to ourselves; of resentment and anger at the world for not fulfilling our desires; of not being able really to love ourselves and to face our inadequacies and aloneness fearlessly. We are all addicted in one way or another to the preservation of our ego. Some people manifest this addiction – and all the fears and neuroses it brings with it – in an external way, through addiction to something tangible; while others internalise it and become afraid of the dark, or of being attacked. Strength and personal courage are needed to break the addiction, for it demands opening ourselves to the unknown, to trusting that we will be safe, and to loving ourselves unconditionally. *See also Anorexia, Liver, Obesity, Stomach and p.88.*

Adrenals: The primary function of the adrenal glands is to produce adrenalin, which regulates the heartbeat and blood pressure in response to perceived life-threatening situations. Perceived life-threatening and actual life-threatening situations may not be the same thing, for the body will immediately respond to stress and tension as being life-threatening, even if we think it is not. This shows the seriousness with which the body deals with stress. The adrenals sit on top of the kidneys, which are known in traditional Chinese medicine as the seat of fear; hence their relationship to balancing the effect of fear during stressful situations. Adrenalin is released when we are in an excited state, for stress can be stimulating and creative as much as it can be destructive and damaging. Exhaustion or related problems will arise through accumulated stress and having to face the 'fight or flight' syndrome too often. A quieter, simpler and less self-centred lifestyle will help restore the balance. *See also p.40 and p.90.*

AIDS: With this condition the immune system becomes deficient in helper T-cells and is unable to protect us from infections, such as pneumonia and cancer. AIDS is known to be caused by a virus transmitted through sexual fluid or the blood. It is intimately connected to the thymus gland (as the place which makes the helper T-cells), which is also connected to the energy of the heart. *(See pp.18, 40, 78.)* The fluid system (which is the means of viral transference) in the body corresponds to the emotional energy; the blood in particular to the heart or to love, and semen to the caring and creative energies. So here there is an indication that the emotional system is out of balance and unable to express itself freely, making it weak and vulnerable to invasion. Research shows that the AIDS personality appears to have a tendency to suppress negative emotions such as anger and fear, and to practise denial: denial of feelings and actions, as well as denial of the reality of the immediate world being experienced. This suppression and denial can cause tremendous emotional pain and blockage; it also directly refutes being able to love and accept ourselves fully as we are. The effect of AIDS is that we are no longer able to protect ourselves. Our inner strength, normally fortified by our love and acceptance and our desire to live, is undermined and weakened. Added to this, there can be a confusion about sexuality and the power of the sexual energy. The sexual experience can be one of the most emotionally uplifting and even spiritually inspiring events as the sexual energy emerges from the seat of the base chakra, the source of our spiritual impetus. However, if this energy is misused, if it is used purely for self-gratification and indulgence, it can then turn against itself. Having no pure expression, it may become diseased, or ill at ease. *See also pp.41, 91.* It is also important to note that as we are out of balance, so our earth is also out of balance. This imbalance then weakens both the human and the planetary immune systems, creating vulnerability to stress and disease. AIDS may well be a symptom of such disease, in which case it is not so much that any one individual has AIDS but that it is something we are all affected by. It thus becomes a global issue demanding awareness, sensitivity and compassion.

Allergies: including **Hay Fever:** These are similar to asthma, but with allergies the reaction is in the eyes, nose and throat, rather than in the lungs and chest. An allergy is an overactive response by the immune system to an outside antigen; this response results from an inner cause. What are we really allergic to? Or over-acting towards? What is really causing the irritation and strong emotional response in our bodies (sneezing, eyes watering, maybe a desire to cry)? These are all responses of the emotional system, the release of suppressed emotions through the reaction. Allergies tend to indicate a deep level of fear, maybe a fear of having to participate fully in life, or of being free of props and having to be self-sufficient, since having an allergy is also a way of getting extra sympathy, support and attention. Are we using our allergy as a means to get love? What is it that we are really avoiding confronting or dealing with? What is it that we are so afraid of letting into ourselves, that we are reacting so strongly against? Is there something that we so mis-trust that we have to push it away? *See also Asthma.*

Alzheimer's Disease: This condition is related to **Dementia,** in which we slowly lose our memory and other intellectual functions, leading to confusion, the inability to hold clear conversations, unawareness of our surroundings, a childlike mentality, fits of violence and other incapacitating aspects. Medically, it is caused by nerve cells in the brain becoming blood-starved, degenerating and dying, and the brain actually being damaged. The causes indicate that both emotional (fluid) and mental (soft tissue) factors are involved, and it is taking place in the head: the centre for abstract awareness and relationship with the higher states of consciousness. It would appear from the causes that there is a withdrawal of the life-giving emotional input (blood), resulting in deep mental trauma. This trauma may be an intense fear of what lies ahead in old age and death, so much so that there is a reversion to childlike behaviour and a shutting down of present-day awareness as a way of ignoring the future. This state has also been described as a preparation time, a period when we can play out our fears and fantasies while living in a semi-alive state, a state that can even border on keen awareness and understanding. Then, when death comes, it is not so fraught with the unconscious terror that was being felt prior to the onset of cell degeneration. Love and support are essential.

Amnesia: Personal pain can be so great that the mind deals with it by completely burying it. Most of us experience memory loss to some degree or another, especially the memory of uncomfortable times in our childhood. Recall is difficult and not always pleasant, as it can mean confronting those hidden and dark areas of our psyche. However, complete amnesia indicates a desire to have another go, because the old life got too much to bear, and was overwhelming in its overt or covert implications. There may be tremendous guilt or shame from the past, actions whose occurrence we are trying to ignore, or people and situations that became separated from reality.

Anaemia: This is caused by a shortage of iron in the blood which may be due to an inadequate diet, an excessive loss of blood, pregnancy or stress. In these cases it is important to recognise and look after our own needs. The blood represents love and related emotions, circulating from the heart throughout our body (our world), so this state is related to a lack of substance, strength or depth to our love (see *Blood*). This undermines the entire blood system, resulting in an inner weakness where we are not able to love even ourselves, let alone anyone else. This may be due to a belief in weakness, that we do not think we are capable of truly loving; or to a belief that we are unworthy of love; or to a fear of feeling love.

Angina: This literally means a tightening or choking sensation, most commonly associated with a pain in the region of the heart, when the demand for oxygen is greater than the ability to supply it. It can be seen as a strong warning from the body that our attention is not where it should be. Instead of exerting outwardly, being very busy, probably stressed and ignoring the inner world, more time should be given to loving and nourishing ourselves and our loved ones. The lack of oxygen implies we are giving too much to others or we have nothing left to give and need to emotionally replenish ourselves. *See also Heart.*

Ankle: The bridge between our being and the ground, the ankles allow our energy to flow downwards and find roots, a much as they allow energy to come upwards from the earth. If that energy is being blocked then it will get held in this area. Our ankles are also our support system – the mental and emotional structure we have built that we rely on to carry us through our lives. When that support structure is threatened or damaged then we have nothing to hold us up and our lives can collapse, just as the whole body gives way when the ankle collapses. So this area is also where we express our ability to support and hold ourselves upright. A **sprained ankle** is a mental conflict, maybe because our support system is changing or being challenged, because we are feeling ungrounded, or because the direction we are going in needs to change. This is especially true of **twisted ankles:** the energy is literally twisting us round to face in a different direction, because we are unable to continue relying on the ground we are walking on. A **broken ankle** is a much deeper conflict in which the very core energy we depend on can no longer sustain us and gives way. With all conditions there has to be a period of no movement at all, which allows for integration and change to take place. *See also entry on the side of the body affected and pp.23 and 95.*

Anorexia: Both anorexia and **obesity** are very closely linked, but although they arise from the same cause they take opposite paths. The cause is the sense of unfulfilled love and affection, the need for emotional nourishment and unconditional acceptance creating an emptiness inside that is demanding satisfaction. Where obesity is the result of feeding the emptiness in an attempt to satisfy it, anorexia is the result of starving the emptiness in the hope that it will shrink and therefore demand less, or even go away completely so there is no demand at all. When suffering from anorexia we continue to see ourselves as being overweight, even when we are already quite thin. In other words we still see our emotional needs as being too great to live with. Anorexia can relate to a feeling of being nagged or crowded in upon, and therefore to a desire to prove independence and individuality; it is a feeling of being out of control of events, and then becomes an exaggerated way of trying to regain control. There may also be a desire to retreat from sexual maturity by making the body like that of a young girl. This is usually due to past sexual abuse or trauma, or to deep emotional insecurity. Unconditional love and acceptance are essential. *See also Addictions, Bulimia and Obesity.*

Anus: This is where we let go, release, become free of that which we no longer need. Problems here are connected to holding on or 'holding out', as children often do as a way of getting revenge on their parents. This is also where we dump many of our fears and inner stresses, such as being in an interview when we might have a great smile on our faces but the anal muscles will be clenched tight. The anus is in the pelvic area, so is to do with ourselves in the world and our relationship to the world. How much are we holding back and trying to ignore? What would it feel like if we were able to let go? Can we relax our hold and not need to control events or people?

Apathy: A giving up on life, an indifference, a deep lack of purpose, interest or direction. Apathy may be due to shock, trauma, abuse, lack of unconditional love or other negative situations that have drained any joy or reason for being here. It can also be due to self-dislike, arising from deep shame or guilt. A need to find new purpose and direction is essential.

Appendix: An aid to the immune system, the appendix is a filter connected to the intestinal tract. **Appendicitis** indicates the breakdown of the ability to filter incoming reality, and to protect ourselves from that reality. As it is in the pelvic area it is primarily to do with our relationship to our relative world and our ability to cope with that reality.

Appetite: Our relationship to our appetite rests largely upon our relationship to ourselves and to our being or feeling emotionally hungry or fulfilled. A lack of fulfilment leads to a deep inner hunger, not just for food but also for love, excitement, or other diversions that take us away from facing the real issue: the inner emptiness. A devouring appetite indicates an avoidance of looking within for answers, as if by eating or consuming as much as possible we will find some sense of satisfaction and release. As we become emotionally fulfilled (by loving ourselves more and thus being able to love others), so our appetite can return to normal. *See also Addictions, Obesity and Stomach.*

Arms: Our arms reach out to hug and touch people, sharing the energy coming from our heart; or they hurt by fighting and resisting. They also enable us to express our creativity and executive nature, for it is here that we are able to 'do things'. When there is a holding back of this energy moving through the arms, it will cause muscular stiffness, lack of free movement, pain, tension, or inflammation and swelling of the joints. **Skin irritation** can indicate an irritation or frustration with what we are or are not doing, how we are expressing ourselves, or how we feel about what someone else might be doing to us. *See also entry on the specific difficulty, the side of the body affected, and also pp.24, 67.*

Arteries: These blood vessels are the means for our love to flow *(see Blood)* from the heart to the rest of our body, or from ourselves to the rest of our world. Therefore the arteries are the means we use for the expression of our emotions. Complications or problems arise to do with conflicts in that expression, particularly of love, and of our ability to share with others. *See also entries on specific conditions.*

Arteriosclerosis: This condition involves a thickening, hardening and loss of elasticity in the walls of the arteries, exacerbated by the addition of fatty deposits, narrowing the walls and making them less able to expand. The arteries carry blood, the life-giving and love-giving fluid within us. A thickening of the walls means that less blood can pass through, therefore less love is being expressed. This may be due to repressing or withholding our love; a fear of expression, maybe due to past rejection; a self-dislike that is so intense that it gets projected on to others; or a criticising and arrogant nature that denies the importance of love and becomes rigid, unbending, fixed and opinionated. Obviously a softer, more loving and accepting attitude to life will not only enable a fuller expression, but will also enable others to show their love and care towards us. *See also entries on the side and part of the body affected.*

Arthritis: This condition affects the joints with inflammation, pain and stiffness. The joints give us free and graceful movement, so arthritis is connected to our innermost feelings about the movement we are taking, what we are doing within that movement, or the direction we are going in. There may also be a sensation of the energy pulling back from moving forward, maybe out of fear of the movement, or because we would really rather be doing something or going somewhere different. This state also indicates self-criticism (stiffness), lack of self-worth, fear, anger (inflammation) and bitterness (pain). There can be a sense of being tied down, restricted, restrained and confined; also a developing inability to bend, to be mentally flexible or to be able to surrender. This can reflect a lack of self-trust as well as a hardening attitude towards life. These feelings are about ourselves, but rather than being acknowledged inwardly they are usually projected outwardly towards others. The part of the body being afflicted with arthritis indicates further information; *see also entries on the specific joint and side of the body, Joints, and Rheumatoid Arthritis.*

Asthma: An asthma attack is usually caused by an over-reaction to pollution or an allergy-causing substance, or by an emotional or stressful situation. This causes a difficulty in breathing out. Asthma in children is particularly associated with our relationship with our mother, as seen in the 'smother' mother or one who over-protects her child and does not allow the child to 'breathe' or live for itself; or in situations where the child is left alone a great deal and has to 'breathe' or look after itself at too early an age. Attacks may be triggered by separation from mother or emotional situations connected to her. Asthma in adults is associated with stress: having a dominating spouse or boss, feeling smothered by spouse, relatives or responsibilities, so that we feel we have to breathe on our own without any support. Asthma is known as the 'silent scream', the longing for expression coupled with the repression of feeling; the desire to expand and enter into life is followed by a contraction and an overriding fear. This is seen in the inability to breathe out. There is a fear of expression, of releasing anger, rage or grief, and therefore a build-up of that emotion inside. Expression must be encouraged – especially in children – so that the deeper feelings can be expressed. Asthma is an over-reaction by the immune system so it is important to express any over-reaction of our emotions. *See also Breathing and p.80.*

Athlete's Foot: A highly contagious fungal infection affecting the skin between the toes due to damp or infected conditions. Itching, sores and skin flaking in the toe area indicate mental irritation, something getting under our skin and causing stress, to the point of digging in, creating inner pain. This is the area of our most forward movement, for the toes go first and the rest of us follows. So this irritation is to do with the details and personal concerns connected to the outward direction and movement of our lives, with what lies ahead.

Back: This is the place where we put everything we do not want to look at; like an ostrich we believe that if we cannot see it then no one else can either! Backache indicates a desire to run away from something, to turn our back on it; or we need to get rid of something we are carrying around, to get it off our back. It may also be that we are holding on to energy in a particular area, and releasing this means looking at all the issues it was holding back from our conscious mind.

Upper back: This area is behind the heart, so expresses the back side of the heart energy: anger, resentment, resistance to loving expression, fear or rejection of love. This can be seen in the **dowager's hump,** an accumulated mass of tissue that can be formed by these repressed and frustrated mind states *(see p. 73).* This part of the back is also a part of the shoulders, so the energy expressed here is connected to our confusion and inability to be doing what we really want to. This is the first stage after conception, so here lies our uncertain purpose, our thwarted ambition, our unfulfilled longings to do or be something different. Pain here is to do with the load we are carrying but not acknowledging openly, the hidden load of repressed and negative feelings. Acne in this area is repressed anger or irritation trying to find release. Often this is because we have become separated from who we really are and what our deeper feelings are. Here also we will experience resentment towards someone who is a 'pain in the back'; or we will want to turn our back on someone, thereby turning our heart away from them.

Middle back: This part of our back corresponds to the quickening period in the prenatal pattern *(see p.30),* which means the shifting of our energy from the inner world to the outer one. In other words, here we find either the ability to express ourselves freely and give meaning to our lives, or the blocking of this energy which leaves our outward expression shallow and empty. The energy is moving through this part of our back as it grows in maturity, so resistance here can be a resistance to maturing and even to facing our impermanence. It is a movement from simply being concerned with ourselves to entering into relationship with and concern for others. Within that movement there can be conflict with power or self-identity, where we become either grossly involved in our ego, or so insecure that we are unable to reach out at all. *See also p.74.*

Lower back: This is part of the pelvis, and therefore a part of our support system and moving centre. From here the energy moves downward and out into the world, and upward towards the heart. But this is the back, so it is also where we store the resentment and frustration connected to our movement, direction or social support, that we do not want to deal with. This area is to do with relationships. How often have we 'bent over' to help someone, and how often has that help been returned or acknowledged? It is also closely linked to our sexuality and to repressed sexual energy, and to the first two chakras. When we look at the pre-natal pattern we see how, as the energy moves down our back, it matures until we reach birth at the genitals. The lower back represents this maturity and the various aspects of ageing. Lower back pain may therefore indicate any one of these conflicts: resentment towards others; fear of moving forward in our personal lives; sexual conflict; a feeling of having no support; an inability to share; or a deep conflict with getting older and facing our mortality. *See also p.75.*

Balance: *See Ears.*

Bed-wetting: This uncontrollable and unconscious release of negative emotion (urine) is also a way of getting attention and affection, as the underlying cause may be a feeling of rejection or unworthiness, insecurity or a fear of the future. The urine represents negative emotions that are normally released as they are no longer needed or wanted. The uncontrollable release of this at night, when we are unaware, indicates that the conflict is on a deep, unconscious level. Blaming a child (or adult) as if he or she is doing it consciously will simply create further conflict and inner pain. Loving and showing unconditional acceptance will be much more helpful, as well as enabling the inner fears and insecurities to be expressed. *See also Bladder.*

Birth: This is the most traumatic transition we ever experience, one that colours our ability to cope with moments of transition and change in the future. *See p.31.*

Bladder: Here we release all our unwanted and negative emotions in the urine, so indirectly the bladder stops us from drowning in our own negativity! Bladder infections are invariably to do with that negative energy: irritation, frustration, hurt and anger not being expressed or released normally. What is it that we are holding on to that should be released? As this is the area of relationship, the most common times for such infections are during a honeymoon period, or a relationship conflict or break-up. The honeymoon experience brings up many issues we are not always prepared to deal with, and can spark anger or resentment towards our partner, as if he or she is to blame for what is coming up within ourselves. A relationship break-up invariably means that many emotions are not getting voiced and released towards the ex-partner, but are getting bottled up inside. (This can also apply to children in relation to the conflict between their parents.) These emotions accumulate and cause the bladder to become irritated and inflamed. The bladder also indicates our ability to adapt to situations, as it adapts to being filled and emptied. This is particularly seen in situations that are hard to accept or adapt to, such as a relationship change. *See also Urinary Infections and p.90.*

Blindness: Accepting and integrating our reality is not always easy, especially if it is painful, abhorrent, confusing or abusive. One reaction to this can be to withdraw our sight, to withdraw from the visual impressions that confront us. By shutting down our sight we can more easily ignore what is going on around us, although the feelings will still penetrate. Blindness is connected to not wanting to see or accept the reality of our situation, to 'turning a blind eye', rather than confronting and dealing with that reality. It can also be caused by diabetes, or being so overloaded with impressions yet unable to integrate them that there is confusion and a sense of not having anywhere to turn to. *See also the entry on the side affected, Eyes and p.58.*

Blisters: Although badly fitting shoes or the over-use of hand tools can encourage a blister to form, the weakness in the body is usually already present which then manifests as the blister. This weakness is a mental irritation that finally causes an emotional eruption. In the feet this will be to do with our security, the ground we are walking on and the direction we are taking. The back of the heel, where blisters usually emerge, is to do with the mother: our relationship to mother earth (reality), to the mothering qualities within us, or to our actual mother. Blisters on the hands represent irritation and frustration with what we are doing and how we are handling our lives. This frustration needs to find an emotional release. *See also entries on the side and part of the body affected.*

Blood: The heart is our centre of love, and so the blood is the expression of our love, circulating through our world outwards from ourselves. It is the life-giving liquid that flows throughout our whole being, carrying our emotions and feelings. Any condition of the blood or the blood vessels is directly to do with our feelings or conflicts about love, our ability or not to express those feelings, our desire to withdraw them, an emotional overloading or outpouring. For instance, **bad circulation** resulting in cold limbs can indicate a withdrawal of blood, and of expressing our love into those areas (whether it be the hands or the feet) that meet other people. *See also entries for specific blood conditions, Heart and p.80.*

Blood Clot or Thrombosis: This is literally a clotting or blocking off of the release and circulation of love. It may arise at a time of feeling neglected, abandoned or unacceptable, when love seems to have been taken away or expression is hindered in some way. For it is as much a blocking off from loving ourselves, as it is a blocking of the ability to love others or to receive their love. It is also a congealing of love, which implies a lack of movement and often occurs in the legs, which are our expression of moving forward. This can imply an attempt to hold on to love in the fear of it moving away, or a fear of us moving away from it (as in the elderly dealing with impending death, when it is an expression of the fear of moving forward). *See also entries on the side and part of the body affected.*

Blood Pressure: High blood pressure damages and narrows the arteries, thereby restricting the flow of blood throughout the whole body. It is a major contributor to heart attacks and strokes. High blood pressure therefore indicates a boiling, a rising of emotion, maybe anger or hurt, in relation to love. Unexpressed emotions become bottled up and create the need to sound off before we get too hot or frantic, or before they block off the means of expression (the arteries). It is also due to nervousness and anxiety giving rise to panic, a fear that the love in our lives is not dependable. **Low blood pressure** indicates a withdrawing of energy. As if we cannot stand up for ourselves, cannot cope with the demands of life, we become overwhelmed and so resist full participation.

Boils: These represent an eruption of emotions, such as anger, rage, irritation and frustration. *See also Abscesses and Acne.*

Bones: The bones represent our deepest core energy, the crystalline energy within us, which also corresponds to our highest spiritual energy. The manifestation of our desire to be here, they are the underlying framework upon which our whole being is built. From deep within the bone, at the very core of our being in the marrow, are born the immune cells which are our ability to protect ourselves. *(See p.40.)* A **break** or **fracture** of a bone indicates a deep conflict affecting us on this inner core level. A break implies we cannot continue in our present state as it immediately hinders our movement; instead fundamental change is needed. *See also entries on the part of the body broken.* **Decalcification** (as in **osteoporosis)** implies a loss of intent or purpose, loss of interest and reason for being here at the deepest level. A loss of that which gives strength to the bones, it is a withdrawal of energy, as the reason for living has gone or is being undermined, often occurring at a time of great change. *See also entries on the side and part of the body affected, and p. 15.*

Bowel Problems: These are related to our ability to surrender and let go, to being secure enough within ourselves to be spontaneous. Problems here reflect a need to hold on to and control what is happening. *See Anus, Constipation, Diarrhoea and Haemorrhoids.*

Brain Tumour: A tumour in the brain is the most dangerous kind, as there is no space for it to expand other than by bearing down on the brain itself. A tumour implies a congealed mass of mental energy (soft tissue), and the head is the area of our relationship to the abstract, as well as being the focal point of experiencing our reality (through the senses). A tumour can therefore indicate a deep mental conflict with being fully in the world, of dealing with reality in a comfortable way. It is a statement of withdrawal, of confusion about participation. There may also be thought patterns or attitudes that are stuck and not going anywhere, in relation to the abstract, to the higher realms of our being. *See also Cysts and p.55.*

Breasts: The most obvious and outward expression of femininity, from her breasts a woman is able to nourish and care for others, as well as to appear soft and intimate. However, there is great social conflict with the breasts, to do with being a woman, being a sex symbol, not being taken seriously, not being able to express femininity or womanhood truly, feelings of inadequacy, shame, fear, embarrassment and self-worth. Breasts are worshipped at the same time as women are put down; women are expected to have children as well as to go to work; if a woman does not want children then there is something wrong with her. These are just some of the conflicts facing women today. Added to these are the inner expectations a woman has in being able to be a woman and a mother. The breasts can easily become rejected as the symbol of all these conflicts; they are close to the heart, so deeply connected to feelings of love and to a sense of self-identity and value.

Breast cancer tends to indicate deep mental thought patterns and attitudes, often ingrained since childhood, about what it means in society to be a woman versus the inner personal feelings and conflicts of being a woman; and the freedom to express those feelings. *(See p.81.)* Breast cancer is connected to feelings of self-worth, to being acceptable, and to being unable to express the feminine nature of caring and nourishing inherent in all beings. As breast cancer is on the increase it can also be attributable to the rise in environmental and toxic pollution.

The **left breast** indicates issues to do with the feelings connected to acceptance as a woman, to being a mother, or to how we feel deep inside ourselves about being a woman. The **right breast** is more to do with being a woman in the world, with what is expected of women and with the breasts in a more external form. It can also be to do with shame and self-dislike. *See also Cancer, Chest, and Heart.*

Breathing: The taking in of breath gives life, the lack of breath is instant death. Our breathing mechanism is therefore the symbol for our separate and individual life and complications here are invariably to do with our desire to live, and to feel at ease with life. Being able to breathe deeply implies the ability to take in life, to be fearless and at peace with life, or to be fearless of ourselves, so **deep breathing** is an indication of our ability to give life and strength to our emotions. **Shallow breathing** implies a fear or resistance to life, often happening at times of distress or panic. The shallow breather is also more likely to be repressed emotionally, living life in a shallow and meaningless way. Breathing is a natural rhythm such as that of the seasons, of the tides, of the moon, and of birth and death. Breathing is also the rhythm of taking in and giving out, of contracting and expanding. So difficulties with breathing can indicate a reluctance to give out, to share, to enter into; or a fear of taking in, of absorbing and merging. It is a holding tight to self and a resistance to letting go, to surrendering self into the whole. *See also Lungs and pp.29 and 80.*

Bronchitis: Here the bronchi become inflamed, whether due to pollution, irritation, infection or a build-up of emotion. Their normal job is to bring air into the lungs, so it may be that what is being brought in is causing us to feel irritated or emotionally choked; but equally it may be what is coming up inside that we need to express and get off our chests, something that is causing a restriction in breathing. An inflammation tends to indicate repressed anger or rage or 'hot' emotions, perhaps due to what we are emotionally breathing in, or due to hidden feelings of shame, guilt or rage we have about ourselves. Or we may be feeling emotionally overwhelmed and unable to breathe for ourselves. The bronchi connect the lungs to the outside world, in the same way we need to find a way to share our feelings, however fearful they may be. *See also Breathing, Chest, Lungs and p.80.*

Bruises: A bruise occurs when we hit something. That 'something' is usually static, so it implies that we went into it, not that it came into us. If we are going forward and we hit something, then obviously we are going in the wrong direction, are not looking at where we are going, or should have changed course to avoid the objects in our path. A bruise is a mental pain or anguish, an expression of a livid emotion we are not verbalising, or a direct warning that we are not paying attention to what we are doing and where we are going in life. It may also indicate that the direction we are going in is not the one we really want to be going in, hence we are not looking ahead. When there is a tendency to bruise easily all the time it implies a complete lack of resistance to life, an attitude that we think we are a victim and have to suffer whatever comes our way. Taking control, becoming the director and making our own decisions is very important here. *See entries on the area and side of the body affected.*

Bulimia: This condition has much the same inner causes as **anorexia** and **obesity,** but its symptoms are a large consumption of food followed by vomiting. In this case the self-dislike is so great that vomiting is preferable to being healthy, it is a way of confirming the self-disgust. To eat and then to throw up contains no joy, so there is obviously a deep depression and desperation. Unconditional love and acceptance are essential, as is the need to facilitate a release of the desperation rather than the release of the food. *See also Addictions, Anorexia and Obesity.*

Bunion: This is a bone deformation near the big toe. Being bone, it is indicative of a conflict on the core level within. This bone weakness is said to come about from wearing the wrong shoes, but a healthy foot can wear most things without damage. Instead the shoes are simply bringing to the surface a weakness that is already there. This area of the foot corresponds to the time just a few weeks after conception *(see p.28)*, and indicates a weakness of commitment to really being here. It usually arises at a time of entering into a relationship with a very dominant partner, parent or spouse. The preference is for the partner (or parent) to make all the decisions, thereby releasing responsibility for us to have to make any decisions ourselves. This puts us in a nicely passive state, where our lack of commitment to being here is eased and free of responsibility. *See also p.96.*

Burns: When we suffer from these something is burning us up inside, both mentally and emotionally (as a burn involves both soft tissue and fluids). Deep pain, anger, grief and other 'hot' emotions may be being repressed and ignored. For instance, burning our foot may indicate a tremendous or burning pain within about a move we have made, or a decision taken about our security, that triggers a strong or hot emotional response. The means of burning can also be indicative: being burnt by boiling water indicates an even stronger emotional input (someone or something has burnt or is burning us emotionally), whereas being burnt by hot wood or another hard substance implies more of a mental or spiritual burning up. *See entries on the side, part and function of the body affected.*

Bursitis: This is an inflammation or swelling of the bursa, a small sac that minimises friction at the joints. The joints are our means for fluid and graceful movement, so when they become damaged in any way it indicates we have become rigid and unbending in our expression. The bursa minimises friction, so it enables our movement to stay easeful and effortless. Inflammation indicates intense irritation and frustration, making the movement become a painful effort. *See entries on the side and part of the body affected, and joints.*

Buttocks: This is the part of the body that we sit on, where we bury the stuff we don't want anyone to see, where we hold back our private tension and anxiety. By clenching the buttock muscles we can still keep a smile on our face and pretend that everything is OK! This is our seat, which in a positive sense implies finding our place in the world, our seat in life, but may also mean we are not too happy about the seat we are presently sitting on. *See also p.76.*

Callosities: These are thickened and hardened areas of skin. The skin is soft tissue or mental energy, so this indicates a thickening and hardening of mental thought patterns or attitudes, creating a 'stuck' state where no energy is moving. This is an accumulation of mental energy that is going nowhere but which is not being released. *See entries on the side, part and function of the body affected.*

Cancer: Where TB was the main illness of the nineteenth century, so cancer is the main one of this century. The immune system becomes suppressed and ignores abnormal body cells, which are then allowed to proliferate unchecked. It would appear that cancer cells are developing in our body all the time but are normally destroyed by the immune system. So what is it that changes this process so that the cells start becoming malignant? Is it because the body has grown so used to the abnormality in terms of thought patterns and attitudes that it does not recognise the difference when those thought patterns become malignant?

Cancer appears to be the result of many years of inner conflict, guilt, hurt, grief, resentment, confusion or tension surrounding deeply personal issues. It is connected to feelings of hopelessness, inadequacy and self-rejection. It has even been called 'acceptable suicide'. It is as if the deeply embedded resentments or conflicts eventually begin to eat away at the body itself. There is also a theory that cancer cells are cells that have become isolated from other cells, through the breakdown of the inter-cellular communication pathways. These isolated cells then produce more isolated cells. This theory tends to reinforce the premise that cancer is based on self-rejection, conflicting or disharmonious attitudes towards a part or parts of ourselves that we do not want to deal with.

The cancer 'personality' that has emerged over years of research is one that is very loving, supportive and kind but simultaneously repressing personal feelings; long-suffering, but with a low sense of self-esteem. When we give so much to others we are often putting their needs ahead of our own and are not giving to ourselves – not really loving or honouring ourselves. The cancer-prone personality is the 'rock' in the family, the one who carries all the problems but never complains. Fulfilment is found by looking outside rather than inside, due to the misbelief that others are right and we are wrong. This very benignness to others can then become malignant in ourselves.

Cancer often follows tragedy or the death of a loved one, especially one who was the object of our attention. That loss simply enhances a sense of hopelessness and worthless-ness. The death may have happened some years previously, but all the feelings of loss, emotional pain, guilt or fear became bottled up and thus remain alive inside. There is an inherent loss of purpose with the death of a loved one, a deep sense of despair. This inner pain is often hidden behind charity or voluntary work, a giving to others when we need to be giving to ourselves.

Inner worthlessness can be related to a lack of unconditional love in childhood that normally assures us of our value and worth in the world. It is also related to feelings of failure and incompetence, with no sense of self-accomplishment. By constantly making other people the object of our attention, we manage to ignore this inner pain. A tendency then arises to repress feelings, especially anger, and deny them expression. Because of this intrinsic imbalance it makes it harder for us to deal with the cancer when it does develop.

Obviously there are external factors that can increase the susceptibility to getting cancer – carcinogens are present in our lives in many forms. However, the inherent personality weakness or repressed mental attitudes described above, can be a major contributory factor as to why some of us will get cancer and others will not when faced with the same conditions.

The function and the part of the body that develops cancer is usually directly connected to the hidden attitudes and unconscious mental patterns involved, as there is a natural tendency to reject the part of ourselves that is causing us pain or conflict. *See entries on the part and side of the body affected.*

Candida: A yeast infection that develops in warm and damp conditions, such as in the vagina or the intestines. As this is an infection it implies we are being infected, or affected, by something from outside. Such infections are normally kept under control by bacteria. So what is it that changes the conditions? In the vagina it suggests unexpressed conflicts to do with our sexuality or sexual activity. It may be that issues are arising due to our relationship that we need to look at, or that something to do with our partner is causing great irritation or heated feelings. Perhaps previous issues of abuse have come to the foreground. In the digestive system, Candida suggests our diet or lifestyle is out of balance, we are feeling insecure or threatened by something that is eating away inside us. Something is upsetting us that we are not admitting. We need to pay attention to balance, purification and lifestyle. *See also p.91.*

Canker Sores or Mouth Ulcers: These are sometimes caused by herpes, and are most likely to occur during or after a period of intense stress, trauma or illness. The mouth is the gateway to the body where we take in food, water, air and reality. This is where we first have to deal with what is coming in and to begin the breakdown and assimilation process. Canker sores are a way of showing us that the reality we are taking into ourselves is causing us to react with distress and irritation. The mouth is also where we express ourselves, so conflict here can be to do with our feeling free to say what we need to. *See also Herpes, Mouth and p.61.*

Cataracts: A cloudy area appearing in the lens of the eye that progressively distorts vision. Losing sight implies a withdrawal of energy from that function and organ – an inner desire not to see what lies ahead. This state usually occurs in the later years of life and is often connected to a growing fear of becoming old and helpless. The future image we have of ourselves is not always one that we want to see, even if that image is not yet a reality. It can be enough to realise that we cannot bend over so easily any more, or cannot remember things that only happened a short time ago. The future can look pretty bleak at these moments. Cataracts are also common in undernourished people, often from Third World countries. Here the lack of inner as well as outer nourishment is starving their souls and bodies. The future looks very bleak so it is not surprising if there is a desire to retreat from it, to put a veil between self and reality. *See also entry on the side of the body affected, and Eyes.*

Cerebral Palsy: This condition involves partial or complete muscular spasticity caused by brain abnormality, often occurring at birth. The muscle is the soft tissue, and here it becomes overactive and does not cooperate with other muscles, producing disorganised or spastic movement. This implies a deep confusion about being here. This may be a karmic pattern that the child is bringing with him or her; but none the less unconditional love and constant reassurance of that love can ease the trauma and mental paralysis.

Chest: The chest is connected to our sense of identity and the inner part of our being. Here lie our heart and lungs, those organs that enable separate life to function. When we talk about ourselves it is the chest we point at when saying 'I'. We 'put on a good front' to meet the world, hiding our real feelings and vulnerabilities inside. *See also entries on separate chest conditions, and p.77.*

Children's Illnesses: We all get these, and in fact our parents try to make sure we get them! This is the body's way of building strength and resistance. It is also the child's need for time out, for extra love and attention, often coming at a time of difficulty at school, or parental conflict that the child feels insecure in dealing with.

Cholesterol: Small amounts of cholesterol are essential for the nervous system, but we do not need to take it in directly from food as the liver can make cholesterol from other foods. High cholesterol levels in the blood cause fatty deposits that can lead to a narrowing of the arteries, possible heart attack and so on. Most cholesterol in our diet comes from fatty and rich foods, especially meat and dairy products. These foods represent self-indulgence, prosperity and comfort. Self-indulgence is a false idea of giving to ourselves, for in truth all we are giving is extra damage and risk, rather than a real gift. This illusion of indulgence is the illusion that we love ourselves. If we really did love ourselves, then we would not put ourselves at risk! Eating high cholesterol (which often also implies over-eating) is actually a way of denying ourselves life and enjoyment. It is a 'live now and pay later' attitude. *See also Arteriosclerosis.*

Chronic Fatigue Syndrome or **Myalgic Encephalomyelitis (M.E.):** Usually occurring after a virus attack, M.E. can last for years and includes muscle fatigue, mental exhaustion, headaches and emotional weakness. Indicated here is a loss of purpose or direction, of desire for life, as if all the wind has gone out of our sails. It can mean a deep fear of life, of taking responsibility, of coping with demands. The illness becomes a safe place to be, a retreat from action and confrontation. This illness seems to be growing in response to the increase in the pressure to succeed, resulting in a fear of failure and a loss of control.

Circulation: The blood is our love energy circulating throughout our world from the heart, the centre of love within us. Poor blood circulation therefore indicates an emotional withdrawal from the situation we are in. We are pulling back our emotions, maybe to protect them, or because it is too painful to have them so active. Bad circulation usually affects our legs (the emotional direction we are going in, the emotions we are standing or relying on), and our hands (what we are doing emotionally, how we are expressing our emotions, our desire to stop doing this). These are the active and most external parts of ourselves, so this is a withdrawal to the inner levels, a withdrawal from full emotional participation in our world. *See* *also entries on the side and part of the body affected, and Raynaud's Disease.*

Cold Limbs: *See Circulation.*

Colds: Who gets one and when? And who doesn't get one and why? These are important questions, for when a germ or virus takes hold and affects us it is because our immune system is not strong enough at that time to deal with it fully. 'Catching a cold' usually occurs when we need time out from what we are doing, when there are emotional issues bothering us that need to be released, or when the relationship between our mind and body is not in harmony. A cold reminds us of crying; the same watery eyes and wet nose, the same sniffing and sense of despair, the same need to be loved yet also to be alone. Is there something we would really like to be crying about, but are not admitting? As a cold can affect both the chest (body) and the head (mind), so it can also occur when we are putting too much energy into one and ignoring the other. *See also p.60.*

Colitis: This is an inflammation, that may or may not be ulcerous, of the colon. *(See Colon.)* An inflammation implies an irritation, frustration or irritable emotional state, and here that is related to accepting and digesting the reality that is taking place around us, the events that are happening, or the relationships we are involved in. For the colon is concerned with absorbing and dealing with our relative world. An ulcer occurs when this irritation has become so intense that it is finally eating away at us, gnawing at us internally, demanding change in our attitudes. *See also Ulcer and p.85.*

Colon: The colon is the area where we finally absorb and integrate what we have taken in from outside. From here the waste is removed through the rectum. The colon is the first place in our body to feel tension, so any changes in the reality around us that are hard for us to digest will be felt here. The action of peristalsis, waves of muscular contraction, keep the contents of the colon moving along. In other words, there is continual mental activity involved in sorting, absorbing, assimilating and integrating our world. **Cancer of the colon** is now one of the top three forms of cancer experienced in the West. There is no doubt that the average Western diet, consisting of large quantities of

animal products, refined grains and sugar, is a major contributory cause of colon cancer, as these foods are hard to digest
as well as lacking in nutrition. However, if we consider the fact
that many people in the West are also not very happy with their
lives or with the world around them, that there is a constant
searching for more – more pleasure, more possessions, more
satisfaction – then perhaps it is not surprising that the major area
in our body where we absorb and digest our reality is subject to
becoming cancerous. Here we are, living a life fraught with
stress, striving to achieve our goals, yet when we do achieve
them finding little real joy there after all. In the meantime we are
constantly eating indulgent foods as a way of rewarding
ourselves for all our hard work! Our poor intestines are having
to deal with both our mental and emotional states and stresses,
as well as the foods we pour into them. And we take little time to
relax or be at ease, little time to find the joy that is deep within us.
See also Cancer and p.85.

Coma: This kind of persistent unconsciousness can last for
weeks or even years, usually as a result of an accident. Under
natural circumstances in this state we would probably die –
certainly we would within a few weeks – but now we have the
medical capability to keep ourselves alive almost indefinitely.
For the first few days it is important to talk to the individual in
the coma and reassure him that if he wants to die then he is free
to do so, and that it is safe and loving for him to awaken if that
is what he wants. This is obviously a state of choice, where both
life and death can be beckoning, and the choice may depend on
the individual's relationships and experience of life. It is
important for the family around the individual to work with
their own feelings and to support the individual in whatever
happens, even if that means that he dies. When the coma
persists beyond a few weeks, we need to look at the family and
people around the individual to see to what extent their own
fears of death, or unfulfilled longings are keeping the life going.
It is even more important now to reassure the individual in the
coma that it is safe to die, as his own fear may be keeping him
here, even though there is barely any life present.

Concussion: Usually due to accident or injury, concussion
causes unconsciousness and temporary departure from the
body. This is a direct way of stopping any movement forward

and can therefore create the situation in which we have the space to reassess our lives and see what direction we really want to be going in. Concussion is also an indication that we may be living too much in our heads, that we are too 'spaced out' and need to come back to earth and deal with reality a little more. It is a severe knock on the head to remind us of where we are and what we are meant to be doing!

Conjunctivitis: This is an inflammation of the membrane covering the eye and the inside of the eyelids, which causes weeping eyes and swelling. Inflammation indicates irritation and frustration; here it is directly to do with what we are seeing and how we are feeling about what we are seeing. The result is a mental swelling, mental heaviness, as well as an emotional outpouring similar to crying. It may well be that we would rather not be seeing, would rather be blind to the vision, as what we are seeing is giving us pain. This does not cause complete blindness, just blurring, which indicates that it might be to do with what we are seeing on the more subtle levels, rather than the obvious ones. *See also Eyes.*

Constipation: The inability to have regular, easy bowel movements indicates a muscular holding on or clamping down. This state is very common in the West, often associated with a lack of fibre or bulk in the diet. *(See Colon.)* A lack of muscular movement indicates that we are trying to control events, to hold on to them for fear of letting go. This implies a lack of spontaneity and 'go with the flow' attitude, a desire to control due to insecurity, for if we are feeling very insecure then we will want to hold on to everything we can. This can also be seen as not taking our seat, in other words not coming into our own sense of security and personal power, that then allows space for all things to be as they are without us interfering. Relinquishing control implies a deep trust and ability to surrender to what is. *See also p.86.*

Coronary: *See Heart.*

Cough: An irritation in the throat or lungs can make us cough. This usually indicates that we are trying to clear ourselves of something, whether it is getting 'something off our chest' or releasing tension in the throat. An irritation is associated with frustrating and irritating attitudes; when there is a discharge, there is also an emotional release. A persistent cough implies that we are not recognising or releasing the irritant in our lives, which may well be an aspect of ourselves that we are not happy with. It is also indicating that we are choking on life, are not at ease with our reality. A cough can arise when what we are taking in is causing us to want to cough it back out again. *See also Bronchitis, Lungs and Throat.*

Cramp: Taking place in the soft tissue, the muscular system, cramp indicates a clamping down or mental seizure, a holding and blocking of energy or thought patterns that are expressing anguish and inner pain. Normally energy moves through the muscles without interference, but here there is so much pressure that the muscle area affected becomes cramped and stuck. Is it to do with our direction or standing (legs), or to do with what we are doing and expressing (arms)? *See also entries on the side and part of the body affected, and p.17.*

Cuts: This involves the soft tissue (flesh) and often the fluids as well (blood). A cut indicates a deep mental pain that is cutting through and causing a wound within. When this wound bleeds it implies there is an emotional outpouring, one of emotional hurt or confusion. The cut may simply be a warning that we are extending ourselves too far, or moving too fast in the wrong direction. But it may also be a sign of deep conflict, as if there is a chasm inside us that is full of upsetting emotions. *See also entries on the side and part of the body affected.*

Cystitis: Inflamed Bladder. *See Bladder, Urinary Infections and p.90.*

Cysts and Tumours: Soft tissue corresponds to the mental energy, so a cyst or tumour is a gathering together and solidifying of mental patterns or attitudes that have been accumulating unconsciously over a period of time. This can represent a whole process of mental thought patterns or attitudes that we build up at certain times in our lives, maybe in defence to protect ourselves against something, or to avoid confronting an issue within ourselves. These attitudes then begin to stick together, to congeal and to become a hindrance to our moving forward, for they are actually already past and useless but we are still holding on to them. *See also entries on the side and part of the body affected.*

Dandruff: This is the dry, white flaking of the horny layer of the skin, usually on the scalp. Horny (meaning hard) is the key word here! Peeling skin indicates an accumulation of excess mental energy trying to get free – dead mental patterns and attitudes no longer needed. The scalp is our abstract as well as our mental and thinking centre. So dandruff tends to imply that there are mental thought patterns or ingrained attitudes we can well do without, we can let go of, for they are actually obsolete although we are holding on to them. They are creating a layer of dead energy surrounding our abstract centre.

Deafness: A withdrawal from hearing, or of taking in the reality around us, deafness is often a response to not wanting to hear what is being said, or is the result of vocalised trauma, and is associated with conscious as well as unconscious choice. It is also a way of creating a barrier between ourselves and our world. Deafness says, 'Leave me alone, don't bother me'; it is a great defensiveness, as much as it is a way of avoiding our own feelings of pain or anger. *See also entries on the side of the body affected, Ears and p.59.*

Depression: This involves a deep inner sadness and longing for life to be different, a conflict between the ideal and the real, between who we would like to be and who we are. There is no doubt that there is a chemical or hormonal imbalance that can cause this state, but the cause of that imbalance may be found in deep, underlying attitudes and emotional issues. How much pressure to succeed did we experience when we were children? Have we experienced life-changing events, such as war, that make ordinary life seem meaningless in comparison? Have we lost our purpose and reason for living, maybe because a loved one has been lost? Depression clearly demonstrates the relationship between mind and body, for as the mind becomes depressed so the body loses its vitality and healthy functioning. Deep relaxation and a reconnection with our purpose are essential.

Dermatitis: This is an inflammation of the skin. The skin is the part of us that meets the world first, and it therefore reflects many of our inner insecurities and fears. An inflammation is an irritation or repressed anger trying to find expression. This anger may be as much towards ourselves as towards others. Dermatitis is a way of reacting if someone is 'getting under our skin', irritating and upsetting us, or if something we have done is now causing us frustration. It is also a way of creating a barrier between ourselves and others, thus avoiding contact. *See also entries on the side and part of the body affected, and Skin.*

Diabetes: This is due to a deficiency in insulin, so that the body cannot utilise the sugars in the bloodstream. The result is the inability to maintain sweetness. Excessive sugar in the blood causes excessive sugar in the urine, leading to a sense of inner sadness as the sweetness is lost and flushed away. If we are diabetic we may be starving in a sea of sweetness, thinking that none of the sweetness is available to us. This can give rise to anger and resentment, to thinking we are unloved when really there is too much love and we just do not know how to deal with it or express it. We may even feel we are being drowned in love. So diabetes is directly to do with balancing the sweetness in ourselves and our world, honouring the love both within and without. It is to do with being able to love others, to give of our own sweetness, as much as it is to do with being able to love ourselves and to receive the love from others. *See p.89.*

Diaphragm: This great sheet of muscle is the dividing line between the upper and lower parts of our being, and helps us breathe. Tension here is due to a resistance to breathing deeply and therefore to taking in life, for when we breathe deeply it demands a surrender and inner relaxation. If we have been holding on for many years to self-control and fear of the consequences when letting go, this is not easy. The diaphragm corresponds to the quickening point in the gestation period *(see p.30)*, the shift in consciousness that moves our energy from awareness of self to awareness of other than self. Here the inner energy can get blocked and repressed on its way out to meet the world. If we are in a situation or lifestyle that does not allow for free expression of inner thoughts and feelings, it is here that they can get held. It is likely that we will also be breathing in a shallow and tight way. *See also Breathing and p.83.*

Diarrhoea: When food moves so quickly through us that we have diarrhoea, the cause is often due to a desire to run away, to be avoiding a situation. Diarrhoea is a way of not integrating the reality that is taking place, whether through fear (as in an animal defecating when confronted with an enemy) or because it is totally unacceptable. This can be seen in the diarrhoea that many travellers experience when in Third World countries: often the experience of poverty, sickness and death can be too overwhelming to absorb. If there is regular, but not serious, diarrhoea (just loose stools), it can indicate a personality type that does not listen; when we eliminate so fast, we do not have time to integrate and assimilate. We need to slow down, listen, hear what is being said before responding, have time to absorb the goodness and nourishment from a situation, as well as that which is not so easily digested. *See also p.85.*

Dislocation: This involves displacement of a bone, putting it out of joint. It means a dis-placement a dis-location, or 'loss of location', a loss of direction and movement from deep inside, a loss of our place in the world. This then puts us out of joint, or stops us moving forward with grace and ease. The bone is our core, our deepest energy, so this indicates a deep sense of imbalance, of confused purpose. *See also entries on the area and side of the body affected, Bone and Joints.*

Diverticulitis: This inflammation of small swellings (diverticula) in the walls of the colon rarely occurs in countries where the diet is high in fibre; when it does occur, it can cause great pain. Diverticulitis indicates that the reality we are taking in and absorbing in our colon is causing us tension and pressure which is then released through creating an abnormality in the mental energy, or soft tissue structure. *See also Colon.*

Dizziness: This expresses itself in a loss of centre, of stability and groundedness. Reality has become overwhelming, and within that we lose our sense of balance and harmony. *See also Ears.*

Ears: The ears are for hearing, so problems in this area are directly to do with that function. Deafness can arise when we cannot deal with or accept what we are hearing, so we withdraw energy from that ability. **Ear infections** can occur when what we are hearing is causing us irritation, emotional upset, conflict and disharmony – literally infecting our hearing. In a child this might be expressing conflict to do with the home environment, or fears and disharmony at school. Indirectly the ears are also to do with maintaining the balance of the bodymind as it moves through the world. This balance keeps us upright and focused, able to be centred and directed. When we lose our centre we lose our balance. This can also happen when we are at odds with what we are hearing! *See also Deafness and p.59.*

Eczema: The skin is the outermost part of our being, the part that meets the world first. Eczema is like a snake shedding its skin – it is the releasing of an outer layer of mental thought patterns (soft tissue) and attitudes, so that a new being may emerge. As it is common in children it indicates that this is something they might have come in with, like an old personality, that needs to be released. It may also suggest a difficulty and frustration in being able to move on and leave the past behind, as the skin does not always peel easily; this frustration can then affect our behaviour and we become irritated or frustrated. It may indicate a sense of being blocked or interfered with, unable to make ourselves and our needs understood. This is also an allergy to the world, a way of saying 'stay clear'; perhaps the reality outside is making us want to retreat even though our real longing may be for intimate contact. Eczema can also indicate a great uncomfortableness with ourselves and the image we are projecting – hence the desire not to deal with it but to withdraw energy and just close up inside. *See also entries on the area and side of the body affected, and Skin.*

Elbows: The elbows allow free movement of expression and creativity, enabling us to put our arms around something (without elbows we would have two stiff poles coming out of our shoulders!), to express ourselves with grace. It is also where we can put energy into what we are doing (elbow grease). Stiffness, soreness or other trauma in this area is therefore a blocking of the energy as it moves down through the arms, maybe to do with fear or confusion about expressing the heart energy or the activity of the doing centre. We might also be feeling elbowed out of the way by someone else, or be trying to elbow our way in, as the elbow expresses quite an aggressive energy that can be used as a weapon. The left or the right side of the body can be indicating different things. *See also entry on the side of the body affected, and p.68.*

Enteritis: This is inflammation of the small intestine, which is where we absorb the nutrients and information from what we are taking in. Enteritis occurs when something we have absorbed, in the form of emotion, thought or feeling, is causing us intense irritation and frustration and is poisoning us rather than nourishing us, but we are holding on to it. The ingested item is turning against us and inflaming us emotionally. *See also Colon, Intestines, and p.85.*

Epilepsy: This is created by miscommunication between the brain's nerve cells, causing one set of signals to become too strong, thus overwhelming other parts of the brain. An epileptic seizure follows, characterised by complete loss of awareness, maybe even loss of consciousness for a few minutes, and sometimes accompanied by violent convulsions. Two-thirds of epileptics show nothing physically wrong with them; with the remaining one-third there is a causal connection to brain damage, head injury or brain tissue infection.

Epilepsy indicates an overloading of the nerve circuit – that what we are dealing with in our lives is too much, making us want to opt out. Yet this sense of being overwhelmed may actually be a result of exaggerating events in our minds. This exaggeration can lead to arrogance, to thinking that we know better than anyone else, for how could anyone else possibly understand what it means to have seizures? Epilepsy is also a cry for attention and love, perhaps due to earlier abuse or rejection. It is a state that sets the sufferer apart, makes him or her different, which is one way of gaining that extra attention as well as reinforcing our sense of superiority. A miscommunication implies a lack of communication, and here it can be seen as a lack of communication between ourselves and our inner selves, that part of us that is secure and loved but which we are out of touch with. Epilepsy takes place in the head, so indicates that there is a tendency to be too abstract or involved in the psychic realms, thus avoiding dealing with relative reality; there is a difficulty in recognising the ground and the world around us as being safe and loving.

Eyes: As our 'windows to the world', our eyes do not just see outwards but also express every emotion and feeling being experienced inwardly. *(See p.58.)* The functioning of the eyes reflects how we see life and our relationship to it, whether it be focusing on the immediate reality and not looking ahead, not projecting ourselves outwardly, which is the introvert nature **(near-sightedness)**; or ignoring the personal and the present in favour of dreaming about the future, being extrovert and gregarious **(far-sightedness)**. If only one eye is affected it is important to take into account the issues related to that particular side of the body *(see p.19)*.

Eyestrain implies we are trying too hard to find answers outside rather than looking inwards for answers and resolution. The more we push or search outside of ourselves, the further away we get from our inner core. If we are experiencing **blurred vision** then it is as if our version of reality is not meshing with the reality confronting us; this indicates a difficulty with focusing, on being clear, and on accepting what we are seeing. For often we do not want to accept what our eyes are telling us. **Blindness** is the extreme version of this condition when, whether due to shock, trauma or inner fear, we withdraw from seeing, withdraw energy from the sight organs, so we are protected from having to deal with the reality being seen. However, the outer darkness of the blind person appears to be beautifully compensated by the world that opens up within, the private but colourful world of the inner spirit.

Astigmatism seems to be related very strongly to parental influence, where the fear or abuse experienced in childhood causes the energy to try to create a different reality, one that is not the same as the one being played out in front of the eyes. **Wide and bulging eyes** are often developed during childhood when confronting rage, anger or fear becomes a normal part of life. The eyes take on the fearful expression, although the child may actually stop registering the fear, as the muscles around the eyes are in a constant state of shock. **Itching eyes** indicate something we are seeing is causing us irritation and we want to rub it out of our sight. *See also entry on the side of the body affected and separate eye conditions.*

Face: This is the place where we confront and meet the world, exposing our inner self. Here we put on a good face, face up to issues in life, lose or hide our face. Through our face we are judged, accepted or rejected. Here also we express our inner fears and insecurities, or we wear a mask and hide our feelings behind it. *See also p.57.*

Far-sightedness: *See Eyes, and Hypermetropia.*

Fatigue: This means weariness with life, inner tiredness because of having to cope or keep going; depression and hopelessness. There is a sense of being inadequate, incompetent and uninterested. It indicates a loss of purpose and direction, a need to reconnect with the inner joy and love of life. *See also Chronic Fatigue Syndrome.*

Feet: The feet are our means to be grounded and solid in the direction we are moving in, to feel secure in our relationship to the world. They are the most outward manifestation of our moving centre, the part of us that moves forward first and furthest. They are what we stand on and rely on for stability and direction. Problems with the feet indicate a conflict with the direction and movement taking place, as well as a lack of security or stability in our world. The feet also have reflected in them the whole of our body (as seen in Reflexology) and our non-physical being (as seen in the Metamorphic Technique). Problems here are therefore connected to our entire being. *(See p.25.)* **Flat feet** indicate a collapse of discrimination, an open vulnerability that sees no difference between what is private and personal and what is public. This may also be an attempt to get grounded, to find purpose, although it actually leaves us more vulnerable than before, *see p.97.* High arches are the opposite of this, where the separation between private and public is clearly marked, if not too much so, indicating the recluse or the genius, often aloof and abstract. *See also entries on the side of the body affected and for separate foot conditions, and p.96.*

Fevers: Something is really burning us up, such as intense anger or indignation, and a fever is the way the body has of releasing this burning. Some 'hot' emotion is erupting, or life has become too hot to handle. Sudden fevers in children may relate to inner conflicts and unexpressed rage or hurt – children have no capacity for intellectually understanding their emotions, so they express them through their bodies. This is also a way for them to have time out, to receive extra love and attention, and to adjust to their rapidly changing reality.

Fibroids: These benign tumours are usually found in the womb. Although not harmful, fibroids can stop pregnancy from taking place. Any soft tissue lump indicates a gathering of mental patterns or attitudes that have been suppressed for so long that they have taken a solid form. In the womb this is invariably connected to our feelings of femininity, sexuality, womanhood, and especially motherhood. There may be accumulated or unexpressed guilt, shame, inner confusion, or past hurt and abuse. *See also Cysts and Tumours.*

Fibrositis: This is a stiffness and pain deep within the muscles, in the fibrous tissue. It can be due to straining a muscle (intense mental strain), or to tension knotting up the muscle (mental tension getting knotted). The condition is indicating that our thoughts or attitudes are in a state of rigidity and anguish, that there is lack of flow through the limbs due to this inner conflict. Is it a mental strain related to what we are doing, or how we are expressing ourselves in the world? Or related to the direction we are going in and the ground we are walking on? *See also entries on the side and part of the body affected, and Pain.*

Fingers: The most outward extension of our hands, the fingers are the part of our doing energy and caring expression that is most out in the world. Damage to the fingers indicates that we may be reaching out too far, trying or doing too much, and need to pull back a little. **Arthritic fingers** indicate a criticism of what we are doing, of what the world is doing to us, or a criticism of others; they can also indicate a desire to be doing something different. Through our fingers we create and express, we touch and we love. The type of tissue involved in the damage is important: soft tissue (a cut or sprain), fluids (bleeding or blistering) or the hard tissue (broken bone or nail problems). *See also entries on the side of the body affected, on specific problems, Hands, and p.69.*

Flu: *See Influenza.*

Frigidity: The inability to give sexually implies a deep inner trauma or conflict. It is experienced as a great fear that we will lose something if we give in this way, when in fact the fear is one of confronting that which we are keeping hidden in ourselves. When this fear is present it indicates a long-held belief in being unworthy or ugly, or of deep shame and guilt. It is often brought on after sexual abuse as a child, parental conditioning that sex is wrong, or a belief that love and sex do not go together. The abusive incident may be buried so deep in the unconscious that we are just left with a desire to withdraw from participation, or to reject sex, without any conscious understanding why. The fear of loss implies the need to control the situation. A deeply loving and accepting relationship can usually provide the framework within which these fears can be resolved.

Frozen Shoulder: *See Shoulder and p.65.*

Gangrene: Usually a result of diabetes or bad circulation, or a hardening of the arteries, when the flow of blood to a certain part of the body stops, gangrene creates dead flesh. Blood flow relates to the circulation of the blood and therefore to the expression or withdrawal of the love in our world. Gangrene can result in having the legs amputated, indicating that the withdrawal or shutting down of love from within is so deep that it completely stops our movement forward. The withdrawal is often through a fear of the future; or caused by a deep lack of self-love which gives us no security with which to move forward. This in turn can be caused by ingrained guilt, grief or shame. The need is for the blood to re-enter, for the love to re-enter our expression, movement, and life. *See also Circulation and Diabetes.*

Gall Bladder: Bile comes from the liver to the small intestine by way of the gall bladder. Bile is bitter and represents that bitterness within us, the resentment, anger and frustration we may be feeling, especially towards another person. **Gallstones** represent this bitter and 'galled' attitude towards others that, over a period of time, becomes hardened and 'stony'. A softened, more accepting attitude will go a long way to helping this situation. *See also p.89.*

Gastritis: This is an inflammation of the stomach which is where we begin the process of digestion, of encountering and dealing with what we have ingested in the form of food, liquid, thoughts, emotions and reality. Here hunger arises, whether it is hunger for food or for emotional nourishment and fulfilment. An inflammation implies an irritation; in the stomach it is a feeling of being inflamed by something that we are absorbing into our system, for once it is in our stomach we have no choice but to process it. So something that we have taken in, or been taken in by, is seriously upsetting us and making us wish we could reject it. Our entire system of assimilating and integrating our reality is upset and makes us feel frustrated and irritated. *See also p.84.*

Gastro-enteritis: This is inflammation of the stomach and the bowels. Here the irritant is even greater than in gastritis, as it is affecting not just the point of entry but also the point of departure, indicating that we are so severely irritated by what is happening that we cannot absorb it but are releasing it, still inflamed. *See also Gastritis.*

Genitals: This area denotes the seat of the sexual energy, of the gonads and of the base chakra. Problems here are closely connected to sexual abuse, mistrust and fear, whether it be fear of another person or of our own feelings and potency. There is an enormous amount of energy involved in this area, as sexuality is very powerful and easily misused. This can give rise to guilt, shame, venereal diseases, frigidity or impotence. It is important that love be present in our sexual experiences, so that our sexuality becomes an expression of our caring and loving qualities. *See also entries on specific difficulties and pp.41, 91.*

Glaucoma: This condition involves a blocking of the drainage channel in the eye so that fluids cannot be released; they build up, putting pressure on the retina and causing deterioration of sight. It is most common in those over sixty. As we grow older, what we see lying ahead of us is not always a very pleasant sight. Our back starts aching so we cannot garden any more; or we find ourselves getting tired very easily and needing an afternoon nap. From being active and vibrant people, we see ourselves becoming slower and more set in our ways. This image can be upsetting and emotionally difficult to accept. We do not want to see what is going to happen to us when we get even older. Glaucoma is a build-up of fluid (emotion) that begins to cause sight problems, starting with a cloudiness and inability to see very far ahead. It expresses the emotional build-up and the desire to see only what is immediately in front of us, so that the future image does not penetrate. *See also entry on the side of the body affected, Blindness, and Eyes.*

Goitre: This is due to over-activity of the thyroid gland, resulting in a speeding up in many of the bodily and mental processes. The thyroid gland is responsible for, among other things, regulating the breathing process (as in hibernation); in the pre-natal pattern it is also connected to conception *(see p.26)*, to the coming in of life and the forming of the body. In other words, the thyroid gland is intimately connected to our desire to live, to commit ourselves to entering into life. If that commitment is weak, then the message the thyroid receives will be confused and uncertain: should it continue to maintain life or not?

This may result in **hyperthyroidism**, in which the thyroid overacts, as in goitre, as if by speeding up the bodily processes it will maintain the ability to be here; this is a stressful response, one that mirrors a stressful or self-centred personality. It also indicates a feeling of choking on life. Deep relaxation is essential. Alternatively it may result in hypothyroidism, in which the thyroid under-acts over a long period of time, as if fading away; this is the hopeless and defeatist personality, when we have little desire to enter in to anything. *See also Neck, and pp.39 and 63.*

Gout: This is the accumulation of uric acid (which is usually removed in the urine) and the formation of crystals in the joint areas. The tissue then becomes inflamed and causes extreme pain in the joints, which are our means of movement and activity. Gout is most common in the big toe, the hands, the knees and the elbows. Accumulating uric acid means that we may be holding on to negative emotions that should normally be released in the urine. This holding on begins to crystallise, fixing us in negative thought patterns and attitudes, making our ability to move and act become painful and awkward. The crystals accumulate because there is not enough blood in the joint areas to carry them away. In other words, there is not enough love getting through to balance and ease the negative (painful, angry or hurtful) feelings. The most common places for gout are therefore in the extremities, the places where our energy is moving into expression in the world; and in the joints of those extremities that allow for free and easy movement. *See also entries for the joint and side affected, and Joints.*

Haemorrhage: The uncontrollable outpouring of blood is often associated with emotional trauma or upset; emotions that have become uncontrollable within and are bursting out. *See also entries for the side and part of the body affected.*

Haemorrhoids: Enlarged varicose veins in and around the anus, haemorrhoids indicate an inner straining and forcing of elimination, as if trying very hard to get something out and away; at the same time there is a holding on. The conflict between pushing and holding creates an imbalance. The veins point to this being an emotional issue, which indicates an emotional conflict between rejecting and pushing away, and yet wanting to hold on and keep the emotion locked inside. This can arise, for instance, in children who are being emotionally abused by their parents (and therefore want to reject), and yet who love their parents and want to hold on to having them there. *See also Varicose Veins.*

Hands: The hands are where we truly express ourselves in the world, the outward manifestation of our inner ability to handle our reality. The hands represent how we are handling the world, how we are being handled, how strong our grasp on reality is, how we are expressing our love, as well as our hate (in the form of a fist). Our hands can express every emotion that we possess, as well as being able to put into action every desire and deed that we wish to do.

Cold hands indicate a withdrawal of emotional energy from participation – either withdrawal in expressing our love and care, or in what we are doing in the world, and how we are handling life. **Hot and sweaty hands** indicate an over-abundance of emotion, such as fear or anxiety, in connection with what we are doing; maybe a fear of appearing incompetent and unable to 'do' what is being asked of us, such as the sweaty hands that happen just before an important interview. This may also be a sign of wanting to hit someone, but feeling unable to express it. **Cramp and pain** are connected to our mental capacity to grasp and deal with reality. Such cramping can indicate our fear or doubt about creative expression.

Arthritis often affects the hands, for how many of us are really doing what we want to do, or really expressing our inner feelings and desires? Arthritis in the hands creates a pulling back, a withdrawal from being able to express ourselves or to have a good grasp on our own affairs. The rigidity and stiffness that develop are also connected to the way we handle the world, to our lack of spontaneity or freedom, to a lack of security in what we are doing. Instead there is doubt and criticism, which hinders the natural flow of the joints. *See also entry for the side of the body affected, Arthritis and p.69.*

Hay Fever: *See Allergies.*

Head: The head is our centre for perception, thinking, abstraction, sensing and experiencing. Here lie our mental powers, our control system for the whole body, as well as the more abstract and spiritual aspects of our being. Any problems in the head are invariably to do with our relationship, or lack of it, to the abstract; to cutting ourselves off from the body; or to the conflict between experience and expression. *See also entries for individual head difficulties, and p.55.*

Headaches: Called the 'silent cry of the overburdened mind,' a variety of reasons may cause a headache:

1. Stress and tension, when we become anxious, strive too hard, and create tension. This is especially so when we are trying too hard mentally to achieve something, or are obsessed with getting ahead.

2. The suppression of thoughts and feelings, maybe because we feel they are inappropriate or unacceptable, or because we do not have the courage to voice them. They get locked inside and have nowhere to go. The headache is the reflex effect of negative emotions, such as worry or anger, causing blood dilation.

3. A sense of self-doubt, failure or self-dislike, giving rise to criticism or questioning that we do not want to hear. We feel boxed in and trapped inside our head, and we do not like what we find there.

4. There may also be related causes from another part of the body, such as an infection or constipation, or we may be feeling a bodymind separation.

In all cases, deep relaxation and an understanding of what is going on will help ease the situation.

Heart: The centre of love within our being, the core of our emotions, the heart is associated to the whole range of feelings from love, compassion and tenderness to grief, loss and fear. We can quite literally feel pain in our heart when it is 'broken', and a sense of expansion and energy when it is joyful.

Heart attacks are a desperate way for the body to show us that we are going out too far, paying too much attention to the material, external and more meaningless aspects of our lives; that we are trying to achieve something that actually has little real value. Are we putting too much energy into intellectual activities, and not enough into feeling ones? Do we trust our feelings? What we are not paying attention to is what is close at hand: family, expressing love, loving self and feeling joy; discovering the more meaningful and important aspects of life that are not dependent on how much money or success we have. Just as the heart is to do with love and compassion, so it can also be associated with the opposite, with hostility and rejection. A coronary can therefore be due to chronic hostility, which we think is a rejection of others but the effect is actually a rejection of ourselves. Heart attacks are to do with how we are relating to and feeling about ourselves – whether we are able to feel love and then express that love to others. They also indicate that we are out of touch with the natural rhythms of life. It is three times more common for a heart to fail on the left side, which represents our more emotional, personal and inner aspects. **High blood pressure** contributes to heart attacks; in other words the repressed anger and strong emotions that boil over in the blood, causing high blood pressure, are also a reflection of cutting ourselves off from the feelings in the heart. *See also p.78.*

Hepatitis: This is an infection of the liver caused by a virus, and it affects the whole body with weakness, jaundice, loss of appetite, fever and abdominal discomfort. The liver is our life-giver, cleansing our blood of poisons and excesses, thereby keeping our emotional state (the blood) in an even balance. But the liver is also where we can accumulate excess anger and poisonous emotions, particularly in connection to our relationships. An infection is an irritation causing inner weakness; an infection of the liver implies that there is a gathering of negative feelings that are causing weakness and hopelessness, maybe due to a difficult relationship or one that is causing guilt, anger and conflicting priorities. *See also Liver and p.87.*

Hernia: A bulge of soft tissue or organ protruding through the muscle wall at a weak spot, a hernia is usually due to the pressure of soft tissue beneath the muscle at a time when the muscle is weak or under-used. It is most common in the abdominal wall, which indicates the inner need to explode. The control of anger and similar mental attitudes has reached a point of exploding or, rather, imploding, as it is not being released outwardly. The abdominal wall protects our inner organs and keeps them in place, so a hernia in this muscle may be due to a desire to keep our world in its place by not allowing the release of anger or other strong expressions. But the repressed behaviour has to find a way out. There can be an accompanying feeling of guilt that we are feeling this way, making us push and strain too far, or try too hard to achieve. The hernia is this mental pushing trying to burst out. *See also entries on the side and part of the body affected, and p.17.*

Herpes: This virus infects enormous numbers of people and stays in the body for life. Even after years of living dormant, the virus can suddenly erupt in sores affecting the mouth, lips and/or the genitals (occasionally elsewhere too). The sores indicate a mental and emotional soreness (as both soft tissue and fluid are involved), an eruption of an inner pain. Outbreaks seem to be closely connected to stress and conflicting situations, especially where we are doing something reluctantly or going against our inner feelings (such as having sex with someone we do not want to be with). Herpes can appear as a result of unhappiness, a lack of self-love, as well as being a way of keeping others at a distance, a 'Keep Out' sign, as the areas where it usually develops are ones of prime and personal communication with another person: the lips and the genitals. This brings the questions of guilt, shame, compromise and self-denial into the picture. *See also entries on the side and part of the body affected.*

Hips: *See Pelvis and p.75.*

Hives: These red and very itchy lumps or weals appear in different areas of the body. They can be triggered as an allergic reaction (what are we really being allergic to?) to a food or other substance, but are made worse by tension and stress. Itching can be a result of feeling helpless and unable to act in response to a frustrating and irritating situation. We may be trying to achieve something that is not happening, stimulating our frustration, or wishing things were different. Or something is getting under our skin and causing intense annoyance. *See also entries for the side and part of the body affected, Allergies, and Itching.*

Hyperactivity: This condition is most common in children when their activity is constant and over-charged. It is usually the child's way of ignoring circumstances around him by becoming so involved in what he is doing that he does not have to pay attention to his immediate reality, perhaps because that reality is not comforting or supportive. It is a way of rebelling against circumstances and feelings that may not be voiced but which are being felt (such as parental fears or inhibitions). The condition is also known to be caused through excess sugar and junk food; food of this nature is often a symbol from parents trying to appease or win over their child, or to replace the love and acceptance the child is lacking – such as giving a child some chocolate when what he really needs is a hug.

Hypermetropia or **Far-sightedness:** This is the inability to focus and see clearly what is near at hand, but the ability to be able to easily see what is far away. It characterises the visionary who sees ahead but has a hard time dealing with immediate day-to-day reality; the extrovert personality who is far more interested in others, in relationships and in external events, than in looking inward and developing self. The cause of this state may well have been trauma or shock that led to the belief that the present is not a safe or loving place to be. By becoming extrovert and by looking ahead we can ignore what is happening, or has happened, close at hand. *See also Eyes and p.58.*

Hypertension: Excessive emotional tension, this is often caused by high blood pressure or intense nervous strain. The cause is deep fear and a lack of trust, a feeling that we are in constant danger and need to be on guard. This may be due to past traumatic experience. Deep breathing and complete relaxation are essential.

Hyperthyroidism: *See Goitre.*

Hypoglycaemia: The opposite of diabetes, this is where there is a low level of sugar in the blood so the muscles and cells become deprived of energy-giving glucose. It is usually found only in diabetics, due to too much insulin or excess exercise, though a milder form is found in people who begin to lose energy if they do not eat regularly. A low level of sugar can be due to giving so much that we have nothing left to give to ourselves. This points to the need to start by loving self, honouring and giving to self, and only then loving and giving to others. It can also arise when there is excessive strain or tension and we deplete the blood sugar faster than we can replenish it. *See also Diabetes.*

Immune System: The body's system of self-protection is essential for fighting bacteria, virus and other potential problems. Without a fully functioning immune system we would die very quickly. The immune system responds to our emotional states, as seen in studies showing how deep grief can dramatically reduce immune strength. Immune cells are first developed in the bone marrow, and then the ones destined to become T-cells are carried to the thymus gland, located close to the heart, where they mature. This close proximity and connection to the heart is not accidental. As we further explore the bodymind relationship we can see how the immune system responds to negative and positive thinking patterns and feelings, especially those in the heart. The brain is also very closely linked to the immune system and certain states of mind can have powerful effects on the biochemics of the brain, thus affecting the functioning of the immune system. *See also p.40.*

Impotence: The lack of sexual drive in a man can be related to a fear of surrendering to a woman, maybe due to childhood abuse. It can lead to a feeling of being emasculated, either at work or at home; or to a deep sense of inadequacy when being asked to perform. It often occurs in reaction to tremendous stress and pressure at work, and then being asked to do the same at home. It can be due to guilt, confusion and fear of loss. Impotence is also a way of gaining power by withholding sexually from a partner who is too demanding or abusive. Great patience and love are needed, as well as deep relaxation and inner acceptance.

Incontinence: The inability to control the escape of urine or stools tends to develop in later years as muscle control weakens, which can also be related to a weakening in emotional and mental control. As we grow older our inner feelings, fears, concerns and anxieties change and we become less able to deal with them; we also feel we are losing control over what is happening in our lives, and that lack of control is reflected in the incontinence. This can be seen in anyone who wets themselves when faced with an uncontrollable situation (even uncontrollable laughter!) Reassurance, acceptance and love are essential.

Indigestion: What or who is indigestible? The stomach is where we take in food, reality, thoughts, feelings and events from the outside to digest, assimilate and integrate into our system. If something is causing indigestion, then in some way or another the reality we are dealing with and taking in is creating upset and disharmony within us. It is a reality that is not compatible with our own. *See also Stomach and p.84.*

Infection: When the immune system is not strong enough to fight off an invading antigen we get infected. It is important to remember that there are many millions of germs and bacteria in the air at all times, but it is only occasionally that we get sick and not everyone around us will get that same sickness. Why? It appears that at the time of becoming infected our immune system is weaker than normal, perhaps due to emotional upset or trauma, family or work crisis, or because we have been stressing ourselves too much and need time to assess the changes. An infection indicates that we are allowing outside forces to influence us and have an effect, so our protective powers need to be strengthened and our inner sense of standing reaffirmed. An infection also implies an irritation or upset, one that has weakened us enough to be open to invasion in this way. What is it that is so deeply irritating and affecting us? *See also entries on specific infections.*

Inflammation: This is a bodily expression of an inner inflammation; we have become inflamed or enraged about something and are expressing it through the body. To inflame means to provoke to a strong reaction, to become red, angry and hot. So what is it that is affecting us in this way? What aspect of our reality is causing us to become red and angry? *See also entries on the part of the body affected, and on specific inflammations.*

Influenza: This condition is due to a virus causing chills, fever, headaches, muscular pain, sneezing and so on. It literally means to 'come under the influence of'. Interestingly it has been found that this virus seems to spread far faster and in a far wider area than human contact and contamination can justify, as seen in outbreaks of flu in remote areas of Alaska where there was no contact with an infected human to start it. So maybe the 'influence' that we fall under is not so much the virus as a state of mind that believes we are weak and helpless, or victims of an external force. For instance, it has often been observed that nurses or people who do not believe they will get sick, do not. Influenza seems most prevalent in the autumn and spring, times of great change, when we have to begin contracting or opening. So it may be that these are moments when we need time for the toxins, emotions and inner feelings to be released and cleared, time to prepare ourselves for what lies ahead. Flu affects our whole body and therefore indicates that our whole being is in need of a cleansing and a rest.

Ingrown Toenail: *see p.96.*

Insomnia: The inability to sleep suggests a deep fear of letting go and surrendering. When we sleep we are in a vulnerable and surrendered state; the lack of ability to do this speaks of chronic tension, fear, anxiety and paranoia. This means that we are feeling as if our ego and our survival are being threatened in some way – understandable if we have experienced some deep trauma such as a rape or robbery. But daily, on-going insomnia indicates a severe lack of trust. The thymus gland is closely connected to sleep, and in turn the thymus is connected to the energy of the heart. So insomnia is related to our ability to love ourselves, to trust love, and therefore to trust life.

Intestines: This is our absorption and integration centre for both food and nourishment, as well as for thoughts, feelings and present reality. Here we eliminate what is no longer needed and assimilate what is acceptable. Anything that is causing us unhappiness, confusion, fear, anger, shame or other such conflicting feelings and thoughts can find a release here and create intestinal problems. *See also entries on specific difficulties and p.85.*

Itching: Literally something is 'getting under our skin' when we suffer irritation. If it is in one specific place, then it clearly relates to that area. If it is all over, it is an irritation that is affecting the whole body, our whole being. What or who is irritating us so badly? What is getting under our skin in such an intense way? Itching can also be an allergic reaction, so we need to look at what it is we may be allergic to, what is being felt so deeply that our response is to want to get away from ourselves or from it, to scratch it out. It may also be that someone else is projecting irritation at us. *See also entries on the side and part of the body affected, and Allergy.*

Jaundice: Usually from a liver disease, drug reaction or blocked bile ducts, jaundice is caused by an excess of bilirubin, a by-product of the liver breaking down aged red blood cells and of excess bile entering the bloodstream. The result is yellow skin and whites of the eyes. As this is to do with the cleansing of the blood system it is therefore connected to a cleansing of our emotions. For instance, it can be an inability to become free of feelings that are debilitating us – we are clinging to something, even though it is doing us no good. It is also to do with excess bile, or bitter emotions, entering our blood. These feelings are actually making us turn yellow, or putrid, from their effect. *See also Hepatitis and Liver.*

Jaw: This bone is essential for eating – for beginning the digestive and assimilative process of what we take in, whether it be food or reality. Here also we hold energy to do with stubbornness and anger, by clenching our jaw. So the energy here is two-way: it affects what we take in as well as what needs to be released. *See also p.63.*

Joints: These enable movement to take place with grace and fluidity. If our joints are locked and unable to move we become stiff, our means of expression becomes rigid and unbending. Through the joints we can express ourselves with ease and adaptability. The joints involve hard tissue, soft tissue and fluids, so problems here can affect us in any one or all of these three aspects. An inflammation in the joints therefore indicates a resistance to or irritation connected to movement – maybe a fear of what lies ahead, or a difficulty with surrendering to it. There is a lack of energy moving through the joints, indicating that we are withdrawing energy from that part of our body-mind. This will depend on the area of the body affected. For instance, the shoulder joints, elbows and wrists all allow us to move the energy from the heart out into our hands, so we can express our caring and loving feelings. These joints also allow us free expression of our creative and doing energy, our handling and executive abilities. A dysfunction in any one of these joints can indicate a fear of expressing that energy, an anger or a resistance to it. *See also entries on specific joints.*

Kidneys: The kidneys enable waste products to be dispersed through the urine, thus cleansing us of negative emotions. Kidney problems can therefore be related to a holding on to old emotional patterns, or to negative emotions that are not being consciously released. The kidneys are also known as the seat of fear, which we can see manifested when adrenalin is released in fight or flight situations. Normally the kidneys release this fear through the urine and maintain a balance. When the kidneys become weakened or damaged, it may indicate unexpressed or unacknowledged fear building up. **Kidney stones** have been described as unshed tears, fears or sadness taking form, becoming solidified; or old issues that should have been released but have been held onto and become form. The release indicates a movement forward into a new state of being. *See also p.90.*

Knees: These are the joints on which we kneel, surrendering to a natural hierarchy or to that which is above us; to the movement and direction taking place. The knees are also our shock absorbers, allowing us to ride the terrain of our world with grace and fluidity; they can be damaged when this terrain becomes too rough. These joints are connected to our humility, our flexibility, as well as being necessary to maintain our position or standing. When the knees give way it indicates a conflict with authority; an inner fear about the movement forward we are taking; or difficulties with being able to stand our ground (as with wobbly and weak knees when we are confronted with a life-threatening situation). When the knees become damaged they are reflecting an inner arrogance, stubbornness or resistance, making progress stiff and painful. Fluid on the knees is an emotional holding against the natural course of events, or an emotional resistance to movement. Soft tissue inflammation or pain is a mental conflict or irritation, an egotistic stubbornness that will not let us surrender or give in. Bone or hard tissue damage is a deep inner conflict and implies surrender on a much deeper level, the surrender of our ego or selfishness, as well as a surrender to the movement and reality we are experiencing. Whether it is the right or the left knee adds further information. *See also entry for the side of the body affected, and p.94.*

Laryngitis: This condition is caused by the blocking off of the vocal cords due to inflammation of the larynx, so that no sound can come out. This is usually the result of great fear (as in stage fright), or maybe because of being told that expressing ourselves was unacceptable or inappropriate – as, for instance, in the child who was 'seen but not heard' – and all the unsaid feelings, especially anger, become locked inside. When trying to express them later there can be a great resistance. Laryngitis can also develop if there is a feeling of shame or guilt over what has already been said, therefore stopping us being able to say any more, or a fear of someone hearing what we have to say. This is an inflamed organ – in other words there is a great deal of hot emotional energy here, all connected to the voice and our expression. The problem is to do with our creativity finding affirmation, becoming free with our voice, and the ability to vocalise our feelings.

Left Side: The left side of our body corresponds to the feminine principle. This means the more intuitive, caring, irrational, inward, emotional, receptive and feeling aspects of our being. It also reflects our relationships with the various women in our lives. This refers to both men and women, as we all contain both masculine and feminine aspects to our nature. *See also p.20.*

Legs: These limbs carry us forward, giving us direction and purpose, as well as stability, solidity and grounding. We stand on our legs, which can mean taking a stand for ourselves; just as we may run from here, either to or from situations. The legs move us forward into the world and reflect all the feelings we might have about that movement and direction. For instance, if we are constantly bruising our legs it would appear that the direction we are following is causing a great deal of mental conflict for we are 'hitting a wall' all the time, thus hurting ourselves. Maybe if we turned in a different direction we would find the walls were no longer there. The legs are the external extension of our moving centre in the pelvis, taking the movement from the inner levels out into manifestation. Each part of the leg has its own body-mind relationship. *See also entry for the side of the body affected, and p.92.*

Leukaemia: This condition is cancer of the blood. Leukaemia often appears after the loss of a loved one, as this form of cancer can be directly connected to the expression of love within us, with the relationship between the heart, the thymus gland and the T-cells. Death of someone dear to us can mean intense frustration with ourselves and a bottling-up of emotions. In particular this is the repression of disturbed or conflicting attitudes towards love, as the blood is our love-giving and life-giving fluid; from it comes our nourishment and ability to love others. If our love or desire for life has been damaged in some way, then our attitude to love can become distrusting, dismissive, alienated and confused. We want to isolate ourselves from feeling anything. *See also Blood and Cancer.*

Liver: The liver deals with excess fats, proteins and sugars, helping to extract them from the blood and then to eliminate them. It is literally our life-giver. It is also known as the seat of anger, a place where anger is stored, for keeping the blood clean can mean having to extract the negativity from it. It is intimately connected to addictive behaviour and especially to the repressed anger of which addictive behaviour can be a manifestation. Liver disorders often give rise to depression, which can be seen as anger turned towards ourselves. Liver sluggishness affects spiritual and inner levels of awareness; then we lose purpose and direction. For the liver gives us life, just as it can harbour our fear of life. *See also Addictions and p.87.*

Lungs: This is the place where we take in separate life, breathe in life; the symbol of our separateness, for when we first breathe we are first considered alive, and when we stop we are considered dead. The lungs are in the centre of the chest, the area of self-identity and 'I', so difficulties here are very much to do with feelings about ourselves, rather than about others or relationships. The ability to breathe deeply is the ability to inhale life. If our breathing is shallow and weak, then our life may be insincere and fearful. *See also Breathing and p.80.*

Lupus: In this auto-immune condition our own antibodies turn against us and start destroying our bodies. This indicates a deep emotional guilt, maybe caused by past shame or abuse: a self-hatred or self-dislike that is so overwhelming that we are unable to forgive or fully accept ourselves.

Lymph: The lymph glands are a part of our immune system as they help purify the blood, keeping it healthy and strong. They also 'clean up' garbage in the body (such as dead cells in the blood) for removal. Their relationship to the blood implies that the lymph glands are intimately connected to keeping us in an even emotional state, constantly purifying our emotions. Swollen glands or blocked lymph nodes can therefore imply an emotional blocking or a denial of emotions, leaving us unprotected and vulnerable to invading poisons, or to the effect of poisonous feelings. *See also entry on the part of the body affected.*

Meningitis: This is infection of the cerebral fluid, resulting in inflammation of the membrane covering the brain or spinal cord, and is usually caused by bacteria or a virus. Infection implies a weakness in the immune system and an inability to protect ourselves. Meningitis implies that this weakness is in the area surrounding the brain, so it may be that we have been under tremendous pressure to perform, to excel in intellectual ways. As the brain is also the governing centre for the entire body, this implies a deep inner weakness that is attacking us at our very source. *See also Immune System and Infection.*

Menopause: When the menopause comes it is often seen as an ending to our femininity, an ending to our purpose for being here as a woman, and therefore a loss of direction and fulfilment. It is a highly emotional time (hence its direct relationship to the blood), particularly to do with our feelings of whether we are still lovable and desirable. Many women can become severely depressed at this time, just as men may do when they retire and find they have nothing to do any more – a time known as the **male menopause.** There is a deep need to find the woman inside, not the one that is just a fertile body but the one that goes beyond procreative abilities; to find a deeper purpose for being here, in other words, to find our spiritual direction for ourselves. Menopause, like retirement, can be a time for discovering freedom, individuality, tremendous change and challenge. It can also be a rebirth.

Menstrual Problems: *See PMT.*

Migraine Headaches: Migraines are usually caused by a lack of oxygen reaching the brain. This can be seen as the life-giving energy being withdrawn from our control centre, so we do not have to deal with the commands, but can ignore our reality and the demands being made on us. This is often caused by a frustration with unfulfilled plans, an overload of information and an inability to integrate it, leading to repressed rage. There is also a sense of something that has to be achieved or done, that is being asked of us, and the fear or resistance connected with being able to fulfil that demand. A goal has to be reached, and the thought of it creates pain. What needs to be looked at here is why there is a desire to avoid demands in the first place. Is it due to a very introverted personality? Or is it because there is a deep feeling of incompetence, a feeling that has been reinforced by not being loved unconditionally? Is it because demands are being made that we feel unable to live up to? A migraine is also a way of taking time out, and of getting extra love and attention. This is especially so with children who may be lacking in love, or who are having the attention they need replaced with sweet foods (sugar can be a physical trigger factor for a migraine). *See also Head, Headache and p.56.*

Mouth: Here is where we first take in substances from the outside, it is the gateway to our inner being for food, water, air, nourishment and reality. It is also the exit point for our feelings and thoughts, through our voice and lips. So it is a two-way area and difficulties here will express either aspect: a resistance to what we are taking in and how that is affecting us, how it may be creating a 'bad taste'; or a conflict with our expression and ability to say what we mean. *See also p.61.*

Multiple Sclerosis: In this auto-immune disease the immune system attacks the mylin sheath surrounding the nerve fibres in the brain. This affects the passage of information between the brain and the limbs through the central nervous system. MS may come and go with symptoms that improve or disappear after 2–3 months (when the nerve repairs itself), or it can develop progressively with cycles of slow degeneration. As this is due to the immune system seeing the body as the enemy, we have to ask ourselves how we may have become an enemy to ourselves. In what way are we not listening to our own needs or following our own purpose? The result of MS is a slowing down and impairment of movement, often with deep tiredness, usually affecting the legs and sometimes the arms as well. This implies a loss of purpose or a sense of being overwhelmed. The ability to express ourselves is restricted, implying an inner withdrawing or holding back from our own feelings. Stress can be a major trigger for episodes when we can lose the ability to stand up for ourselves. Or we may feel overwhelmed by the responsibilities of life and want to avoid them. *See also p. 17.*

Muscle: This corresponds to the mental energy. Muscles enable us to move; they give life, strength and power to the inner core (bone) energy. They represent who we are, as we think so we become, and are formed according to our attitudes and experiences. Problems to do with the muscular system are directly related to mental issues, patterns and behaviour that are being expressed in the part of the body affected. *See also entries on the side and part of the body affected and p.17.*

Myopia or **Near-sightedness:** This is the ability to see close at hand while the far distance is blurred, due to tense and contracted eye muscles. In other words we can deal with immediate reality and day-to-day life very easily, but have a hard time creating a vision of the future, seeing the possibilities that lie ahead, or overcoming fear of what is to come. Difficulty may also be experienced with projecting ourselves outwardly, the tendency is to be introverted and shy. This contracted state might be initially stimulated by fearful or abusive experiences ch as the look in the eye of an enraged or hostile parent) that se us literally to withdraw our sight from what is taking e. The trauma becomes locked in the eye muscles, affecting bility to see ahead clearly. *See also Eyes and p.58.*

These are hard tissue, so they represent our inner core ual energy, manifesting out into the world at our most points. They are often affected when our activity or the world is going through change or upheaval, and we are resisting or having a hard time dealing with that change. The nails are also claws, symbols of aggression.

Nausea: We suffer from nausea when something in the reality being absorbed into our being is creating the desire to throw it right back out again. In other words we are dealing with a reality that is causing great upset, sadness and pain, and we do not want to have it anywhere near us. This can also happen when we have done something we wish we had not, so it is a desire to undo the past. **In pregnancy** this is connected to accepting and being at peace with the reality of having a child, and all the various emotions and conflicts that this reality can raise. *See also Indigestion and Stomach.*

Near-sightedness: *See Myopia.*

Neck: The neck is the bridge between the mind and body, the link that enables movement and life to take place. It corresponds to conception, to the incoming life and taking on of form; as well as to the thyroid gland and the rhythm of the breath. It is through the neck that we swallow those things that give us life: breath, water and food. It is also here that we can cut ourselves off from either the head or the body, becoming either abstract and cerebral, or materialistic and shallow. Through our neck comes our expression from the heart, our voice and our love, and our ability to be free with this expression. A **stiff neck** indicates the inability to see on all sides, like a horse with blinkers on so that it can only see straight ahead. This is a very rigid and limited way of seeing, implying a stubbornness and narrow-mindedness. It may also be a response to extreme stress, causing us to want to close in and limit ourselves. *See also p.63.*

Nerves: The nervous system includes the brain and pathways of communication throughout the whole b constantly receiving and giving information to and fror senses, the feelings and thoughts. The spine is the home central nervous system – all the peripheral nerves come spine to relay information. This system controls all conscious activities. Activities of the unconscious heartbeat, breathing and so on) are controlled by the nervous system. Conscious control over this syste gained through meditation or deep relaxation.

As the nervous system covers such a vast arena of activity and functioning, a breakdown or damage can affect us in many different ways. Basically it is a breakdown in communication between one part of our being and another, whether that be between the brain and a limb, or between a feeling and an expression. *See also entry on the part of the body affected.*

Nervous Breakdown: The inability to carry on, this represents a complete breakdown in communication and the capacity to cope, usually due to great emotional or mental shock or trauma. The implication is that there is a need for time to adjust, recover and assimilate what has happened. A breakdown in communication within us on this level can affect us in many different ways. Deep relaxation, acceptance and unconditional love are essential.

Nervousness: This manifests itself in hypersensitivity to others, indicating a lack of contact with our own inner being. It is actually a very self-centred state, in which we see everything subjectively – only as it relates to ourselves. As such we live in fear of attack and abuse; we are unable to relax and be free of selfish or egotistical attitudes. There is a lack of trust and faith. Deep relaxation is essential.

Neuralgia: This pain from a damaged nerve can be very sharp, shooting along the nerve pathway. A damaged nerve implies that a breakdown in communication within us has caused a deep pain. The energy is not getting through and along the nerve; rather it is getting blocked and distorted, causing intense inner pain. It is important to find where the miscommunication is taking place. *See also entries on the side and part of the body affected and Nerves.*

Nose: This is where we first breathe in, taking in air and reality. The nose is a gateway to our higher mind. Here we breathe, but breathing is not always what we want to be doing, especially when life gets a little overwhelming or difficult to deal with. Then we may develop a blocked nose, narrowing the air passages so that the amount of life able to get in is limited. Here also is our sense of smell and our participation in the smell of life! *See also Breathing, Colds and p.60.*

Numbness: The loss of feeling in any part of the body indicates a withdrawal of feeling, or a withdrawal of energy. This withdrawal may be because expression of this aspect of ourselves was unacceptable and therefore repressed, particularly in childhood *(see p.20);* or because that part of us has been hurt so much that we no longer wish to feel it. It is important to ask which part (and the function of that part) is being affected, for the area of numbness can tell us what is happening: the left or right side of the body, the upper or lower parts, or the limbs. Why are we isolating this area in this way? *See also entries on the side and part of the body affected.*

Obesity: This state is often thought of as the price of success: we are now so successful that we can eat what we want and do not have time to exercise! Food is a wonderful relaxant and is emotionally fulfilling, as it is equated in our minds with love and mother. However, when it is used to replace either of these, used to fill the emotional emptiness within, or to compensate for the success that is leaving us emotionally isolated, then obesity can occur. It puts a layer of fat between the inner self and the world, like a moat protecting us from a fear of exposure, from being vulnerable and therefore hurt; yet it can equally stop us from freely expressing ourselves. Obesity often occurs after a great emotional shock or loss, as the emptiness experienced within ourselves becomes too great to bear. This is the feeling of being empty of meaning or purpose, but our attempt to fill that emptiness actually causes more emptiness. The excess flesh indicates that there is a holding on to fixed mental attitudes and patterns of thought, although these attitudes are actually creating discomfort, if not even embarrassment. Obesity in children can be a reflection of their difficulty with acknowledging or expressing their feelings of security and acceptance; for instance, it can develop at a time of parental divorce or death. *See also Addiction, Anorexia, Stomach and p.84.*

Oedema: A swelling due to water retention, oedema causes puffiness and is most common in the ankles and feet. Fluids correspond to the emotions so oedema indicates a holding on, repression or denial of inner feelings and urges. There is a holding and gathering of emotional energy. The function of the part of the body that is affected adds further information. When oedema affects the whole body it indicates a deep emotionally held attitude, perhaps because emotional expression is inappropriate and is therefore being ignored or denied. For instance, there may be a great longing to walk in a different direction, for our lives to be reflecting different aspects of our being, but we feel emotionally trapped in the direction we are going in, or feel emotionally unable to assert ourselves and bring release. With oedema there is a need to acknowledge and then find expression for these contained and bottled-up emotions. *See also entries on the side and part of the body affected.*

Osteomyelitis: This infection of the bone and bone marrow usually only affects one bone, near a joint. The bones are our deepest core energy, also corresponding to our spiritual energy, and the joints give movement and expression to this energy. An infection implies an irritation creating an inner weakness, an undermining of normal resistance that leaves the area open and vulnerable. The issue is a deep one, not easily reached with the conscious mind, for the bone is well hidden within. This infection is putting into question our life energy and purpose. If this is due to previous damage, then it may be that the original causes of that damage have not yet been dealt with. *See also entries on the side and part of the body affected, Bones, Infection and p.15.*

Ovaries: These are an immediate and direct symbol of femininity, of being a woman and of being fulfilled as a woman. Ovary problems tend to indicate a deep conflict with this aspect of our being, of expressing our femininity, with being or not being a mother, or even conflict in being a woman at all. Do we want to have children? Do we resent the children we already have? Are we at peace with being a woman? Would we rather be a man? Has the feminine aspect in ourselves been repressed or abused? Is our husband/lover rejecting or refusing us? Are we being able to give birth to ourselves? Are we going in the direction we want to?

The ovaries are the beginning and creation of life and they are in the pelvis, which is the area where we can give birth to new aspects of ourselves, where we can find ourselves anew. In this way difficulties with the ovaries represent our own inner conflict with creating and finding our own path. An **ovarian cyst** is a sac full of fluid that forms on or near an ovary and is not usually too serious, but it indicates a gathering of emotional energy, of conflicting feelings connected to the ovarian energy.

Pain: Pain is the body's most immediate way of telling us something is wrong, yet we do everything we can to avoid or remove it. Instead, we should take notice and listen. Invariably a physical pain points to a psychological or emotional pain, a physical ache being an inner ache or yearning, a bruise indicating we are going in the wrong direction or doing the wrong thing with the result that we keep hitting obstacles. Pain brings us into the body, it makes us stop and take rest, it gives us time to see where we need to make changes. If we open, tune into and breathe into pain we will find it softens and eases – tensing against it will only increase it. *See also entries on the side and part of the body affected.*

Pancreas: Here the insulin level is maintained, so that we can maintain the sugar levels in our blood. When the sugar levels are off-balance, diabetes or hypoglycaemia can result. The pancreas is therefore associated with being able to express and integrate love throughout our whole being, as well as being able to deal with the opposite feelings, such as anger, without creating pain. *See also p.89.*

Paralysis: There are different reasons for paralysis, but generally it indicates such a complete withdrawal of energy from moving forward that the movement is actually stopped. This may be due to intense fear of what is happening or going to happen, a fear of the future; or to deep trauma, making us want to stop life so that the trauma cannot be repeated; or to intense self-dislike and distrust to the point where the only surety against wrong action is no action at all. The area of the body affected is important, so *see entries on the side and part of the body affected.*

Parkinson's Disease: This condition is the deterioration of nerve centres in the brain, particularly of the areas controlling movement; it leads to shaking and tremor (usually of hands or head), with decreasing ability to move. The breakdown of inner communication is such that the fear of moving into life with commitment and energy, begins to make the actual nerve functioning deteriorate. Shaking and tremors indicate fear, whether it be fear from the past, or fear of the future; it is expressing a fear of moving, perhaps due to past trauma or abuse, and what that movement might involve. *See also Nerves.*

Pelvis: The whole of the pelvic region, framed by the hips and spine, is our area of communication and relationship. Here we can share ourselves through sex; we can create and give birth, not just to another person, but also to ourselves, giving birth to new aspects and attitudes; from here we can also begin the journey upwards through the chakras to higher states of consciousness. The pelvis is the centre from which we move forward in our lives, whether that means taking a new direction in the world, or discovering the realms of the inner world. The **hips** are the bones that support and enable this activity to take place; they represent that deepest level of energy within us in relation to our movement. *See also p.75.*

Peptic Ulcer: This is an ulcer in the digestive tract. An ulcer is usually considered as being caused by stress, although it is our reaction to the stress that is more important than the stressing factor. That reaction might be anger, aggression, fear or nervousness. The ulcer is an area of rawness in the digestive tract, causing intense pain and upset. In other words, our irritating or frustrating attitude to what is happening in our lives is causing a raw and irritated area, in the very place where we take in our reality and begin absorbing and integrating it into our system. It may also be that what is coming in, the reality we are having to deal with, is causing us intense irritation and pain. *See also Intestines, Stomach and Ulcer.*

Phlebitis: This is the inflammation of a vein, usually caused by infection or injury, in which the blood becomes disturbed and may cause clots. The blood corresponds to our emotional, loving energy, and the veins are the means for this energy to travel out and come back to us from within our world. An inflammation in this area implies that our emotional energy has become hot and inflamed, maybe angry or irritated – that something is infecting us, thereby affecting our means of expression. This infection or irritation is causing deep emotional pain. *See also entries on the side and part of the body affected.*

PMT or Premenstrual Tension: This is mental and emotional tension that arises at or before the onset of a woman's period, usually due to a hormonal imbalance. This is on the increase due to the massive rise of hormones in the environment. The monthly period is a reminder to women that they are living in a largely masculine-dominated world; so PMT brings up issues to do with how we feel about being a woman and our relationship to our femininity. It is often very hard to be a career woman, perhaps to be running a business meeting, and to have a period; the two do not go together easily. We respond to our period with emotional and mental disturbance and reluctance, so something here is disturbing us, making us feel awkward and resentful. Do we resent being a woman? Would we prefer not to be working? What are our deeper feelings about these aspects of womanhood?

Pneumonia: An inflammation of the lungs, pneumonia is usually caused by bacterial or viral infection, involving a cough, fever, shortness of breath, sweating and so on. The lungs are where we take in breath, which is life; without it we die. The lungs are our means for separate life, for here we breathe alone. However, there are times when breathing is not so much fun – maybe when life has become somewhat overwhelming, or there is conflict within us about living our lives for ourselves versus being in a very close or dominating relationship. Then our ability to breathe may become diminished, or we may feel stifled. An inflammation indicates that this area has become hot and angry, irritated or frustrated. So our desire and ability to breathe have become severely affected by our emotions; by our fears of being alone or of being overwhelmed; by our anger towards life or towards our aloneness, and to actually being here; or by our irritation with ourselves. *See also Breathing, Lungs and p.80.*

Pregnancy: Although pregnancy is usually a joyful and enriching time it can also be fraught with hidden worries, doubts, fears and concerns, especially when it is the first time. Many of these fears and uncertainties we try to keep hidden, for society says that happiness is meant to be paramount. But these hidden feelings will find a way out, whether it be through constipation (fear of letting go, trying to hold on to things as they are/were); sciatica (fear of moving forward into new territory and the direction that life is going in); heartburn (difficulty in swallowing the reality of what is happening); and so on. *See also entries on specific ailments.*

Premenstrual Tension: *See PMT.*

Prolapse: This is the displacement or protrusion of an organ, usually the prostate, vagina or bladder. A prolapse indicates a letting go, a giving up, a collapse, a lack of control, for the energy is no longer strong enough to maintain elasticity and the muscles give way. This indicates a mental collapsing, a mental giving up, an inner hopelessness, an attitude which tends to be more common in later years. *See also entry for the part of the body affected* and combine that with this sense of hopelessness, depression, a loss of energy, or a feeling of no longer having any control in our lives.

Prostate: This small gland, connected to the sexual functioning in men, is found close to the bladder. It is related to our sense of sexual power and capability and often causes trouble in older men. How many of us can enter our sixties and seventies feeling at ease and satisfied with our sexuality and performance? Most men feel frustrated, impotent, confused, searching for younger partners or giving up altogether. Our sexual expression reflects our inner feelings, and men of retirement age or older often feel useless, ineffectual and unable to be a full man, as if the purpose for being here is already over. A **prolapsed prostate** immediately puts great pressure on the bladder, indicating the added difficulty being experienced in actually releasing those feelings of uselessness that are building up inside, for the urine is the release of negativity and corroding emotions. *See also Prolapse.*

Psoriasis: The over-production of skin cells can cause a pile-up of dead cells, with a thickening of the skin and raised red patches. This is usually triggered by stress, poor health or a lack of resistance. It is a mental issue, a build-up of mental patterns and attitudes that are already dead and finished with but are not being released, so they are causing problems. *See also entry on the side of the body affected, and Skin.*

Rash: A rash occurs on the skin, the most external part of us that meets the world first. Here there is a reaction to something or someone that we are confronting, causing redness (mental or emotional heat) and itching (frustration or irritation). Who or what is getting under our skin? This can also be caused by embarrassment, maybe because of inner shame or guilt; or by an allergy. A rash is related to the function and area of the body where it arises, so *see also entry for the side and part of the body affected, Allergy and Skin.*

Raynaud's Disease: This condition is characterised by constricted circulation to the hands, ears, nose and feet, creating pallid, numb limbs which occasionally turn blue or purple. This represents the withdrawal of emotional energy (the blood) from the extremities, or from those parts of us that meet the world first. This withdrawal may be due to a fear of expression (fearing it to be unacceptable), to a fear of rejection (from previous trauma or deep emotional hurt), or to a change of heart (the ending of a love affair and therefore of extending out emotionally). The emotions, especially the love energy, are being held back, creating a sense of abandonment and loss in the limbs. We are therefore not fully participating in the world and we need to re-enter and find our place again. *See also entries on the side and part of the body affected, Blood and Circulation.*

Rheumatoid Arthritis: This is where the immune system starts attacking itself, attacking the collagen, which is the connective tissue in the joints, as if it were an invading antigen. It is known that this state worsens when we experience extra stress or tension. Rheumatoid arthritis indicates a deep self-dislike, perhaps due to shame or guilt; an inbred sense of worthlessness or self-criticism; as well as long-held anger, bitterness and stiff attitudes. We are attacking our own selves, and the result is painful and limited mobility in moving or expressing ourselves freely. The joints are our means for fluid and graceful expression, so swelling and soreness here indicate a real difficulty in expressing that fluidity of movement in what we are doing and the direction we are going in. The rheumatoid arthritic personality is one that exhibits unassertive and inhibited behaviour, is self-sacrificing and unable to express strong emotions. That lack of expression then manifests physically as lack of mobility; it turns against itself and finds expression in being inwardly critical and bitter. *See also entries on the side and part of the body affected, Arthritis and Joints.*

Ribcage: This part of our anatomy protects our life-giving organs (the heart and the lungs) from damage. It is bone, so this implies it is the spiritual energy protecting our life here on earth.

Damage can indicate weakness, vulnerability, helplessness, or openness to attack. *See also p.82.*

Right Side: The right side of our body corresponds to the masculine principle. This represents the more assertive, rational, logical, intellectual, aggressive, worldly, giving and dominating aspects of our being. It also reflects our relationships with the various men in our lives. These aspects relate to both men and women, as we all contain both masculine and feminine qualities. *See also p.19.*

Sciatica: This is a nerve pain that starts in the small of the back (it can be due to a prolapsed disc or to a nerve being pinched) and runs down the back of the thigh. Since the nerves are our means for communication between all the cells and parts of the body, here we have a deep pain in that communication connected to the expression of our moving energy as it moves into the world (the legs). In other words, the direction we are going in is causing us a deep inner pain, but it is in the back so it is a pain that we are not consciously wanting to acknowledge; we would rather keep it hidden and not communicate with it, or deal with what it is trying to tell us. Sciatica is quite common during **pregnancy,** often highlighting the inner confusion and pain about the direction life is now going in, for pregnancy can be a joyous experience but beneath the surface there can also be many misgivings, doubts and fears. *See also entry for the side of the body affected, Back, Legs and Nerves.*

Sclerosis: This is abnormal inflammation and/or hardening of body connective tissue, a substance essential to every structure in the body. This state appears to be an auto-immune disease, in which the immune system begins to attack body cells and causes the connective tissue to become damaged. Therefore this is a situation in which we are attacking ourselves, at a very deep and essential level, for if the sclerosis spreads to major organs it can cause fatal damage. An inflammation implies a red-hot or angry energy, where long-repressed fury or rage is coming to the surface; it is an emotional state when sclerosis affects the blood vessels. Hardened tissue suggests a hardening of mental thoughts and attitudes, and here it is actually a hardening of that which connects and therefore creates a wholeness out of parts. It is as if we are only seeing bits of ourselves and not the entire picture, or we are breaking up into pieces, for our attitude has hardened against who we are as a whole. Sclerosis can affect any part of the body, so it is saying that this is a state affecting our whole being, where the need to acknowledge, accept and express what is really going on inside is paramount. Learning to love ourselves is not easy, but essential. When we turn against ourselves in this way it can indicate so much self-dislike, guilt, shame and inner unhappiness that it is eating away at us. *See also entries on the side and part of the body affected.*

Scoliosis: *See Spine.*

Shingles: This illness is usually due to the chicken pox virus reacting in adults as a blistering rash running along a nerve pathway. The nerves are our means of communication within ourselves. Here the nerve pathway becomes extremely painful, indicating a breakdown in communication in the area affected. The resulting blistering rash implies an intense emotional reaction or irritation to someone or something. In adults it can be a cry for attention, to be nourished and nurtured as a child; it may also be a reaction to our living situation and experiencing excess stress. *See also entries for the side and part of the body affected, and Nerves.*

Shoulders: Here is where we carry the burden of being alive, the weight and responsibility of having to create, perform and do. The shoulders are the inner part of our doing energy; it is here that the conflict about what we are doing emerges. Responsibility means the ability to respond, yet how many of us are responding to what we want to do in life? Are we happy with what we are doing and how we are doing it? Are we doing one thing but inwardly wanting to do another? If so, then the energy can get locked in here as it has no means for escape. Ideally the energy should be moving from the heart, up to the shoulders, then down through the arms for expression in the world, but if it gets blocked it will cause pain and stiffness. A **frozen shoulder** means that the shoulder becomes cold and painful, hindering its full use. Are we giving a cold shoulder to someone? Or receiving a cold shoulder? Are we hugging the right person? Are we becoming cold and indifferent about what we are doing, just doing it for the sake of doing it but not because we really want to? This is similar to deep **tension,**

which indicates that we would really rather be doing something different from what we are doing. *See also entry on the side of the body affected and p. 65.*

Sinusitis: This is an inflammation of the mucous membranes of the sinuses, causing blockage, a greenish discharge and pain. The sinuses are the air passages in our head and are related to our more abstract and thinking processes, to awareness and to communication. An inflammation suggests an emotional anger or irritation; the discharge is also emotional (fluid), a release of negative emotions, or a state of being emotionally overwrought. Sinusitis can therefore indicate a deep conflict or release of negativity in the area of abstract activity, of thinking, and in our communication. *See also inflammation and p.61.*

Skin: The largest organ in our body, the skin is composed of millions of overlapping cells that are self-repairing and even waterproof. The skin is soft tissue, so problems are invariably to do with mental energy: how we think other people see us, how we see ourselves, as well as expressing our deeper insecurities, uncertainties and concerns. We blush with embarrassment or redden with anger, as the skin is constantly reflecting our inner feelings. If we are thick-skinned it implies that little can get through to us, whereas being thin-skinned implies that we are very vulnerable and cannot easily hide inside. States such as peeling or flaking of dead skin indicate a letting go of old mental thought patterns, like a snake shedding its skin. **Dryness** implies an emotional withdrawal from the area affected, for there is not enough fluid to keep the skin alive. Skin **eruptions** are usually connected to our feelings about ourselves, a conflict with self-identity and our relationship to others. *See also entries on the side and part of the body affected, Acne, Dermatitis, Eczema, Face and Rash.*

Slipped Disc: A disc is a round, flat structure between each pair of vertebrae in the spine, surrounding a jelly-like substance. In a slipped disc the pressure from the vertebrae squeezes some of this jelly out, lessening the cushioning effect and creating pain on the surrounding nerves. This state is a coming together of all three cell structures: the emotions are involved as there is an abnormal release in the fluid; the mental energy is involved as there is pain in the nerves; and the core energy is involved as the slipped disc is being created through a squeezing or pressure from the vertebrae. This indicates a deep conflict affecting all aspects of our being, arising under the pressure from above. Pressure is the key word here. It may be that we are exerting the pressure on ourselves, in an attempt to do or be something more than we are; or that the pressure is coming from someone or somewhere else, making us feel we have to try to live up to something. It is important to refer to the part of the spine affected to understand this further, so *see Spine and p.72.*

Spine: This is the very backbone of our being, the central channel of our nervous system, blood supply, core and spiritual energy. The spine is in many ways the most important part of the body, for it holds everything together and makes life possible. Problems of the spine are related to a problem in the deepest part of our energy system. **Scoliosis** is a lateral curvature of the spine, most predominant in adolescent girls. This indicates a core level conflict with being here, and especially with growing up and facing maturity. As seen in the pre-natal pattern *(see p.25),* the energy comes down the spine, growing in maturity as it does so. In an adolescent girl the fears and concerns about growing into adulthood can be so great as to distort the energy in the spine. The condition can be accompanied by depression or lethargy, for there is a holding back of energy and a desire not to be here or not to have to deal with anything. *See also Back, Bones, Slipped Disc and p.72.*

Spleen: Directly linked to both the thymus gland and the hypothalamus in the brain, the spleen aids in the production and maintenance of immune cells in the blood. It is also connected to the pancreas for the production of insulin. In other words, this little organ is essential for balancing the blood, and for our personal protection. In order to do this the spleen may have to deal with negative emotions, such as anger, that are in the blood, which can weaken this area if they become overwhelming. *See also p.89.*

Sprains: Spraining a muscle, which usually happens at the ankle or wrist, indicates a mental sprain: a mental strain that can no longer be tolerated. We have gone as far as we can in a particular mind-set and need to see that it is not doing us any good or that it is becoming strained. The wrist and ankle are both joints that allow energy through just before that energy manifests in the world (in the hand or the foot). Are we about to do something that we really would be better not doing? Are we handling a situation in such a way that it is causing us real anguish or strain? Are we moving in a direction that we would be better off not going in? Are we standing on ground that is unstable and mentally disturbing? *See also entries on the side and part of the body affected and p.17.*

Sterility: Is having children what we really want to do, or are there deep hidden fears that are too strong to deal with easily? A fear of procreation can also be associated with a fear of responsibility, of financial concerns, or of past traumas from our own childhood. There are many issues at stake when we discover we may not have children, issues that have to be considered carefully.

Stiffness: Muscular stiffness caused by lactic acid accumulation implies the accumulation of stiff or blocked mental energy. Stiffness is the manifestation of stubborn and rigid thinking patterns, an inability or refusal to surrender, a resistance to moving. Although stiffness often comes after hard work, this is simply highlighting a weakness already present in the muscles. The energy should be flowing smoothly through the muscles, cleansing any lactic acid build-up; if it is not, then we can check our mental attitudes in relation to the part of the body affected. A **stiff neck,** for instance, causes too much pain to be able to turn in all directions and this implies a narrowing viewpoint, the inability to see other ways of thinking, to acknowledge or even yield to others' ideas. **Stiff joints** indicate a deeper resistance, as here it is the bone that is stiff; it is a core level rigidity and resistance to moving forward. The joints enable us to move with grace and freedom, so we should ask ourselves what it is inside that is resisting or being reluctant to such movement. *See also entries on the side and part of the body affected.*

Stomach: Here the process of digestion really starts and it applies as much to digesting our reality, the events and emotions taking place in our lives, as it does to digesting food. If our reality is indigestible or nauseating, then indigestion or nausea can follow. The stomach is emotionally linked to food, to love and to mother. The empty gnawing in the stomach is often the need for love or emotional nourishment as much as it is for food. Stomach problems arise when our reality is in conflict with what we want, or when our reaction to that reality is a negative and acid-forming one. *See also Indigestion, Obesity, Peptic Ulcer and p. 84.*

Stress: This can be both positive in being stimulating and creative, as well as life-threatening in its effect on the body. The stress factor itself is actually less important than is our reaction to it: how we react to situations, events, feelings and difficulties is what causes the stressful effect in the body. Rather than blaming external situations for our state, we need to look within ourselves and question our reactions, motives and attitudes. Deep relaxation is essential. *See also p.5.*

Stroke: This can be caused by high blood pressure; or a brain artery can be narrowed and constricted, a blood clot can stick in an artery, or an artery can rupture, seriously damaging brain tissue and activity. All these causes are related to the circulation of blood, and the vessels that the blood passes through. So the means (the arteries) we use for expressing our love and receiving love from others have become narrowed, constricted, repressed. Strokes invariably occur in later life, an indication that there is within us a growing resistance or bitterness about love, maybe because a loved one has died and our love is literally being constricted. A stroke is also a way of trying to hold on and keep things as they are, a resistance to the process of events, especially ageing. The fear of old age and death makes us want to stay fixed in one place so as to avoid further change. Strokes are fairly common when an elderly person is moved into a nursing home, away from the familiar surroundings and normal means of expressing and receiving love. The constriction is so great that it can cause death or paralysis, indicating that the inner pain of loss or repressed emotion is such that there is an equally strong desire to no longer be here to have to deal with it. *See also entries on the side and part of the body affected.*

Stuttering: A fear with being clear about what we have to say, often caused by dominating and authoritative parents, criticising and controlling, or telling us that we are ignorant and don't know what we are saying. We need to relax deeply and learn to trust our own feelings and to love ourselves as we are. *See also Mouth.*

Sweating: Excessive, unusual sweating is usually a sign of releasing fear or similar emotions, related to the part of the body where it is happening.

Swelling: This may be a simple swelling, as happens when we are bruised or inflamed. It tends to imply an emotional resistance or holding back of our feelings. The swelling is a gathering of liquid, a gathering of emotions that are being held on to as they may be inappropriate to express or we are fearful of them. It is also a way of our protecting ourselves, so here we can ask what it is we feel the need to be protected from? When swelling becomes more serious it may be oedema. *See also entries on the side and part of the body affected and Oedema.*

Tears: The free flowing of tears is the free flowing of our emotions of love, pain, fear, joy, hurt and compassion. Blocked tear ducts indicate a blocking of this free expression, maybe due to being conditioned to believe that crying is 'only for babies'. It is important to allow free expression to take place from deep inside, or the repressed feelings can build up and cause physical problems. Crying is our way of releasing that build-up, of allowing the emotional energy (the tears) to be free and therefore to be healed. When we cannot cry it is much harder to find the repressed feelings, to release them, and thus to bring about healing and resolution. *See also p.59.*

Teeth: The teeth are like a gateway through which our reality must pass, for the mouth is where we take in that which feeds, sustains and nourishes us, whether it be food, liquid or feelings. However, we also take in that which is not always so pleasant, in the form of the reality that is going on around us. When that reality is unacceptable it can have a rotting and decaying effect on us. The teeth are the hard tissue, the core energy of our being, so as they begin the breaking-down process of what we are taking in they respond to the feelings inherent within that. They are a part of the means we have of talking, of giving life to the emotions and thoughts we have within us, of expressing all of our being into the world. When we are feeling deep conflict or guilt about what we are saying, the teeth and gums can show this. They are also a means for expressing aggression, as when we clamp down on something. So what is it that we are reacting to in this way? *See also p. 62.*

Tendons: These consist of connective tissues that join the muscles to the bones. This is soft tissue, so it is the mental energy that is connecting to the core spiritual energy to allow full movement and expression to take place. Here we can see a direct bodymind link when we think of how rigid tendons can reflect rigid tendencies! If our mental energy is stiff and rigid then we are usually unbendable, and our soft tissue will reflect this and become equally rigid. Hence we might become more stiff as we grow older and as our attitudes become stiffer. Pain in the tendons implies a deep conflict between what we think we should be doing or where we think we should be going, and what our inner voice is saying we want to do. For the mental/tendon energy is going one way, while the inner core/bone energy wants to go another way. *See entries on the side and part of the body affected, and p.17.*

Testicles: The male sex glands are naturally subject to all the fears, insecurities and doubts about being a man; about sexuality and sexual preference; about ability to perform and impotence. In a tight situation we may feel we are being held by the balls by someone, especially if it is a powerful woman. Are we being taken over, becoming powerless? Losing our masculinity? Difficulties here imply that we need to look deeply within ourselves for hidden feelings about our manhood.

Throat: This is where we swallow our reality, where we take in life through breath, food and water. And this is also where we release our feelings from our heart through our voice. A two-way bridge, the throat is the cut-off point between the head and the body. The swallowing or taking in of substances ensures the body's survival, although not everything we have to swallow is nourishing. When it is not, when we are having to swallow a reality we do not want to, we may find our throat becoming inflamed and sore, trying to close down or cut off our physical reality. This can also happen when we repress anger or rage and the emotion gets caught in our throat. If we are not saying what we really want to say, or there is some conflict in our expression, then our throat will feel the repression. **Strep throat** is one of the most common forms of throat infection, and is caused by streptococci bacteria. An infection implies an irritation and holding back of energy. Is it feelings we are not expressing? Or is the reality around us causing intense frustration and conflict that we do not want to swallow? The throat also represents conception *(see p.26)*, the taking in of life, so difficulties here can reflect a deep conflict with accepting our existence. *See also p.63.*

Thrombosis: *See Blood Clot.*

Toes: The toes are the part of us that goes forward into the world first, and as such they also represent our head (as seen in Reflexology). Toes curled under can indicate a withdrawal from moving forward, a pulling back from entering life, as well as an attempt to grasp and hang on to life, maybe through chronic insecurity. Toes curled up indicate an attempt to be escaping from life, a pushing upwards into the more abstract realms away from the earthly ones. Crossed toes indicate a great confusion in the direction we are going in, or any sense of inner clarity and freedom. *See also p.96.*

Tonsils: A part of the lymph and immune system, the tonsils act like filters, monitoring what goes down the throat; in this way they filter our reality. **Tonsillitis** often emerges at a time when the reality being swallowed is causing an intense irritation or fear, which becomes too overwhelming for the filter to be able to work efficiently. Then the tonsils become inflamed, expressing inner anger and frustration at what is happening. This is often the case with children who do not necessarily understand what is going on and have no control over events – they just know that they are not happy with what they are having to swallow. The removal of the tonsils simply means that we have to swallow our reality uncensored and deal with it in another way inside. *See also Throat and p.63.*

Tumours: These are soft tissue lumps formed in different parts of the body, which are usually harmless unless in the brain. A tumour represents mental thought patterns and attitudes that have been ignored and not dealt with for a long time, or are no longer appropriate; so they have begun to form a congealed mass – have begun to solidify. *See also entries on the side and part of the body affected and Cysts.*

Ulcers: Open sores appear either on the skin or in the membrane, as in **peptic ulcers**. An ulcer involves both the soft tissue (mental) and fluid (emotional) energies, and indicates a growing aggravation or irritation. Something is gnawing at us, eating us up, making us bad-tempered, raw and irritated. This may be our reaction to events such as stress, a reaction that is upsetting and insistent, as the event itself is neither positive nor negative. *See also entries on the side and part of the body affected and Peptic Ulcer.*

Urinary Infections: Inflammation of the bladder or urinary tract **(cystitis)** creates pain on urination and the desire to pass frequently, although there is little release. The urinary tract is where we let go of our negative feelings, maintaining a balance in our system by doing so. An inflammation implies a buildup of anger, resentment, irritation or other 'hot' feelings. This indicates we have an excess of negative emotions to the point where the urinary system is unable to deal with them in the normal way. So although we want to urinate, little is released. This part of the body is in the pelvis, the area where we can move forward into new aspects of ourselves and which is also concerned with relationships. So we may well find that this inflammation is due to a lack of expression of negative feelings to do with relationships (it has been found that 80 per cent of cystitis cases occur at a time of relationship break-up), as well as the fears and conflicts to do with moving forward on our own and giving birth to ourselves, separate to the relationship. *See also Bladder and p.90.*

Uterus: This is the womb, the part of us that symbolises our femininity, our womanhood and our ability to create; it is the inner sanctum that is warm and secure and can bear new life. Problems here reflect the problems we can be feeling in relation to these aspects of our being. How do we feel about being a woman? About having or not having children? Is there deep shame or guilt, or maybe betrayal? Have we lived up to the image that our mother instilled in us? Does our husband or lover find us attractive as a woman? Do we find our femininity over-burdening and hard to deal with? Are we aggressive and dominating? These are just some of the questions we need to ask ourselves if there are uterine problems. Are we holding ourselves back? For this area is in the pelvis, from which we can give birth to new aspects of our being and move forward in ourselves. *See also Cancer and p.75.*

Vaginitis: This is an infection of the vagina, similar to Candida, with a heavy, foul-smelling discharge. Normal conditions in the vagina maintain a balance with any invading bacteria or virus. So what is it that changes, or weakens, allowing this virus to take hold? The vagina is where all our feelings about our sexuality emerge: our guilt, uncertainties, fears, shame, abusive memories, conflicts and confusion. An infection of this nature tends to arise at times when one or more of these emotions are present, maybe stimulated through an intimate relationship. Intimacy can trigger many feelings related to memory or fear. Candida is a way of saying, 'Stay clear', because we need time to assimilate what is happening. The foul-smelling discharge is the release of negative emotions, the release of built-up fears or angers that are buried in the tissue of the vagina itself. *See also p.91.*

Varicose Veins: Enlarged veins, these are usually found in the legs. The blood represents the circulation of love in our world and the veins are our means for expression. In the veins the blood is on its way back; having shared our love, it is now coming back to the heart with the love it has received from our world. Varicosity can indicate a deep emotional conflict directly related to the conflict of being able to love and nourish ourselves, and to being able to receive love from both ourselves and others. This will relate to the function and area of the body affected. Because the legs are the most common place, the implication is that the direction we are going in or the ground we are standing on is not giving to us emotionally – it is confusing and blocking our emotional movement. Common during pregnancy, varicosity can indicate the fears associated to having a child, of sharing our love with another person who is dependent on us, of losing our individuality and suddenly becoming a mother, of maybe even becoming unlovable or losing our ability to love at all. This is very closely connected to the legs as they are carrying us in the direction we are going in, towards birth, and that direction represents the fear we wish to avoid. *See also entries on the side and part of the body affected and Blood.*

Venereal Disease: Here there is a need to look closely at what we are doing with our sexual energy. A venereal disease implies a dis-ease or unease with the energy in this area – that there is a confusion or distortion. Sexual energy is extremely powerful and important; when taken lightly or misused it has a tendency to backfire, to become diseased, giving us an opportunity to see what it is we are doing that is out of harmony with the natural flow and balance of this energy. *See also pp.45, 91.*

Warts: A viral infection in the skin causing excess cell production creating a hard lump, usually painless unless walked on. A hard lump is an excess of mental patterns holding together, and here they appear to be associated with self-dislike and the belief that we are ugly and unlovable. This belief weakens the system, allowing a virus to take hold. If we believe we are ugly then our body will become ugly; it simply reflects our inner attitudes. If we do something we don't like or feel ashamed about, or are doing something we want to but feel we are unworthy of, then warts might appear on our hands. When the situation is resolved, they can disappear. *See also entries on the side and part of the body affected.*

Wrist: The wrists give graceful and fluid movement to our expressive and doing energy. *(See p.24.)* **Arthritis** here indicates a critical attitude towards what we are doing or what is being done to us by others, as well as a desire to withdraw from what we are doing. A **break** or **sprain** in the wrist indicates a deep conflict with expression, either expression of love from the heart outwards, or of the creative and doing energies. This can also be a withdrawal of energy from what we are doing and how we are being handled. Wrist problems may be an expression of hopelessness – that we feel we are not capable of doing something. The fall or break then stops us from having to do anything. **Pain** may also be repressed energy concerning something that needs to be done, but which is being held back and not acted on. *See also entries on the side of the body affected, Arms and p.68.*

CHAPTER 7

The Healing Relationship

Letting go of our suffering is the hardest work we will ever do.
It is also the most fruitful. To heal means to meet ourselves
in a new way – in the newness of each moment where
all is possible and nothing is limited to the old. STEPHEN LEVINE,
Healing into Life and Death.

A s we learn the bodymind language we can come to recognise the patterns in our bodies, what those patterns are trying to tell us, and how they manifest in our lives. In so doing it soon becomes obvious that there is something deeper going on when incidents, illnesses or accidents continually repeat themselves. Recognition is not so hard, once we penetrate the language and symbols being used. However, recognition alone is not always enough to change the patterns, as they are well embedded in our unconscious. For real change to take place there also has to be integration.

Integration can occur in many different ways, whether it be through meditation, visualisation, prayer, counselling, body-work, or through the experience of serious illness. Understanding the bodymind language opens the door for us to start working on this deeper level, to begin acknowledging, accepting and loving who we are, as we are, complete with whatever we find buried within us. In accepting what we find, we can begin the healing process. A healing relationship develops as we recognise the role we are playing in our own state of wellness, recognise what we need to do in order to become free of limitations, and as we integrate the changes that take place as a result of that recognition; in other words, as we bring awareness and love to all aspects of our being.

This does not deny the very important role of medicine; rather it seeks to work with whatever means of medical or complementary intervention we may choose, so that the healing can take place in a complete way. There are many times when the use of drugs or surgery is necessary to save our lives and to provide us with relief from suffering. Free of that suffering, we can have the energy to work more deeply with ourselves. However, removing the symptoms does not equate to a cure. To heal means to become whole, to unite that which has been separated, to attain a wholeness of body, mind, emotions and spirit; whereas to cure means to eliminate or remove a problem, it does not look to the whole, but deals only with the affected parts. If we change the surface by dealing with the symptoms but we make no shift on the inner levels, then we may be subject to experiencing those symptoms, or others like them, over again. It is also possible that we might not be able to eliminate or cure all of the symptoms, as in cases of terminal illness, but that need not preclude or deny the inner healing that can take place.

Healing and wholeness come from the same root: to heal is to become whole. So what is it that is missing in our wholeness? The recognition of what is missing, as well as the integration of the resulting balance, allows a new freedom to emerge, the freedom of movement into new states of being. This is not always dependent on being physically cured, but does imply that we become whole within ourselves.

One of the drawbacks of medical intervention is the level of dependency it has generated. We tend to mistrust the idea that we can heal ourselves, become worried if we do not have sufficient medication, or believe that as long as we get a prescription we will get better. However, most doctors will admit that it is not themselves, or even the prescriptions, that are doing the real work. All that they can do is to provide the environment in which a cure can take place. Ultimately, the power to get well, to be healed, lies within each one of us. We have to want to get better, to be prepared to work on many different issues in our lives, and to change or loosen our fixed patterns of behaviour. Then we can work side by side with whatever forms of medical or complementary therapy we feel we need.

When we first become ill we usually experience fear, hopelessness, shock, anger, resentment and grief – depending on the severity of the illness. Our body is fragile and vulnerable to sickness or pain, and death is absolutely guaranteed at some point. Yet we are never prepared to confront these issues in our lives, we have not been taught how to deal with the emotions and feelings that arise. Most of us live in a state of denial, becoming indignant or even outraged when illness, accident or death happen to us or to our loved ones. When we do fall sick and we are confronted with our own suffering and mortality we have no place to put our feelings, no way of coping with such intensity. It is important at this time to find someone we can talk to, whether it be a relative, friend, priest, doctor or counsellor – someone who understands what it means to be sick and to possibly be facing death.

We are confronting the fear of impermanence, the fear that arises when our separate existence, and particularly our ego-centred existence, comes under threat. The fear is of the future for we know that the future is going to hold sickness, pain and, at some time, our death. Rather than confront and accept these issues, we prefer to hold on to the past, because even if the past was painful and traumatic, we came through it intact so it is safe. By holding on to it and keeping it alive within us we avoid living in the present, for the present implies there is a future, and we would rather ignore the future as it is life threatening. In this way the past begins to fester and rot within us. For instance, the guilt we have been harbouring for twenty years should have been released all that time ago, but as it wasn't it is finally beginning to manifest on the physical level. But if we now let our guilt go, what are we left with? We are left with a void, with the future, with the unknown. Holding on to the guilt has given us a reason for being here, a reason for being as miserable or critical as we are. Without it we have to confront our own emptiness. We have to confront our fear of losing what we think we are, a fear of being without, and open ourselves to becoming what we can be when we are free.

Love is a letting go of the fear. In other words, love and fear cannot co-exist. Where love is expansive and all-encompassing, fear is contractive and exclusive. It is not possible to feel fear and to love at the same time. So if we are experiencing a fear of loneliness, fear of rejection, fear of loss or fear of emptiness, then the only way to overcome these fears is to grow in love, primarily towards ourselves. When we can really love ourselves, we can freely love others and they can freely love us; we do not then need an illness or something similar to facilitate the receiving of that love.

Some years ago I was flying from Philadelphia to Dallas. It was late at night, and as there were only a few of us on the plane we each took a row of seats and settled down to read or sleep. As we came near our destination we unexpectedly hit the tail end of a tornado and the plane became like a feather in the sky, rocking and rolling, with the luggage falling in all directions. Jerked out of my sleepy consciousness as the oxygen masks came down, and sure that we would not survive, I mentally prepared myself to die. It felt OK – that if my time was up then I was ready. Then suddenly the thought hit me that if I did die then I would not be able to tell the people whom I loved that I loved them. It was a devastating moment, and left me in a state of shock at the power of such a thought. At almost the same time I also realised that I was about to be sick, and then the plane managed to pull out of its roller-coaster and we headed towards an airport somewhere south of Dallas.

It was another four days before I got home and had a chance to assimilate what had happened. Over the following few weeks I not only wrote or spoke to the people whom I loved and told them that I loved them, but I also realised that acknowledging my love for them was not enough. I first had to find my love for myself. I had had a profound experience: in confronting death I had confronted love. It was an experience that had shown me the depth and power of love as being so strong that it could hold me back from being ready to die. But as I was integrating the realisation that ultimately love is everything, that it is the underlying energy of all life, at the same time I discovered that deep inside I did not trust love. Past experiences, childhood pain and rejection had all accumulated inside me and formed a deep mistrust of the love that I was now opening myself to. Here I was, experiencing the glory and overwhelming power of love, and yet I did not trust it!

I found that in order to love myself I had to open in a way that was painful, full of sad memories and emotions that hurt. It took quite a while for me to heal the wounds, to resolve the mistrust, but my vision of the power and the depth of love saw me through. I remember a day when I was quietly meditating and I saw my whole life in front of me, from the very beginning with all its difficulties, pains and traumas. And I saw that throughout it all love had been there, love had actually been supporting and holding me even in those most hurtful times. I was finally able to trust it.

To love ourselves may first mean needing to forgive ourselves. We usually think that it is other people we need to forgive, for surely it is the hurt we have experienced through them that has caused us to be so fearful. Yet in reality we know, deep inside, that we are fully responsible for everything that has happened to us; our own guilt or shame are there if we look closely enough. We may translate this as a need for revenge, resentment or anger, but ultimately it is towards ourselves that we are experiencing these feelings. No one can make us angry or can hurt us – it is our reaction that is the anger or the hurt. And that reaction is within us. So then we can ask ourselves how much of our illness is a self-punishment. Are we ready to release the need for revenge, so that the illness can also go? Are we ready to forgive ourselves, deeply, inside, so that we may also forgive others? Are we ready to love ourselves as we are, guilt and all?

As we develop our awareness and become able to acknowledge our inner fears, angers or repressed emotions, we need to find a way of bringing these feelings to the surface so they can be dealt with. From acknowledgment has to come release and resolution. However, it is not always necessary to tell the person who we still feel angry with after all these years have passed, that we still feel angry; we do not even need to release the anger at all. We can actually resolve it within ourselves, transforming the energy into a more constructive and positive power. Anger is simply energy, and energy can be used in any way we choose. I remember seeing this in John, whose bitter and resentful feelings about his father were choking him up, causing deep distress. However, his father had been dead for some years, so there was no way to vent these feelings on him personally. As John began to acknowledge his feelings and recognise the depth and power of them, he was then able to integrate the energy they gave him and to use it for forgiveness for both himself and his father. From being a passive and repressed person, often subject to colds and chest problems, bowing under the weight of his father, John was able to emerge stronger and more energetic, and even became physically taller.

To start the healing process we have to look at whether we really want to get better, for it is not always a simple matter. Many of us will prefer to take a pill than to confront our own anger, or will want surgery more than we want to deal with changing our behaviour. When confronted with the potential for wellness through a particular cure we may find we are withdrawing, or even refusing to go ahead with the treatments. We have to want to get better more than we want the familiarity and lifestyle patterns of being sick. But there can be hidden reasons for our sickness that actually create a reward for us, and these will hold us back from being able to heal. It may be that we are paid lots of extra attention or love when we are ill; or thinking that the illness now makes us a 'real' person. It can be that our disability has become a companion and there is a sense of emptiness at the thought of being without it. Maybe our illness has become a safe place to be, something to hide our fears behind. Or perhaps it is a way of making someone feel guilty for something that has been done to us; it can equally be a way of punishing ourselves, or a way of avoiding our own guilt. And it may be that we really do want to opt out. For instance, intense physical pain can be a reflection of intense mental pain, as seen in cases where physical pain has been relieved by drugs, only to be followed by a nervous breakdown or even suicide.

One way to find our hidden reason is to ask ourselves if we could imagine being well again, and how that feels. We need to do this in a quiet and relaxed way, going deep inside, and being very honest about what we find. I remember working with one multiple sclerosis patient who constantly said she wanted to walk again; but when asked to imagine herself being able to do so, she could not. Most especially she could not imagine herself being without her wheelchair. Deep inside, issues to do with being dependent on others in order to receive their love were stronger than her ability to love herself. So we have to be honest. Do we want to be well, to be free, to have nothing to complain about? To have no specific reason why people should pay us attention? Can we really see ourselves without our difficulty? And if not, then what is our pay-off in being ill? How would we feel if someone offered us a cure? Many of us remember times of sickness as actually being times of happiness because we received so much love. Are we prepared to do without this? So often the major issue at stake with being ill or being healthy is to do with loving ourselves, about feeling lovable for who we are without having to be something 'special', about being in touch with ourselves enough that we want to live for our own sakes, not because of someone else or because of what we get from others.

There are also positive side-effects of illness, such as the time away from responsibilities and demands that enables us to be quiet within ourselves. It may mean we can do things (like taking a holiday) that we would not normally do. And more importantly, especially if we are facing death, it can mean we might be able to express our deeper feelings, like love and caring, more easily. It is just as important to recognise these positive issues and to give them expression, as it is to work with and release the more negative issues.

To move from a state of sickness to one of wellness and healing takes great courage, fortitude and honesty. It also takes hope, which means being active in our healing relationship, rather than passive. We have a tendency, especially in the West, to sit back and just let God or a doctor do it all for us. However, having hope means working with God or the doctor; it means being willing to help ourselves. Becoming hopeless implies a giving up, a depressed and helpless state, one in which we just take whatever pain comes our way, one in which we have become a victim of circumstances. It is a loss of faith and a loss of meaning. It is the belief that nothing can help, therefore we stop doing anything that might help, and eventually nothing can help.

Being hopeful, on the other hand, implies a desire for a bright future, a belief that things will change; it is a state of deep faith. Improvement may not begin until there is this resolve that recovery is possible. It is known medically that those patients most likely to heal quickly are the assertive, persistent ones, no matter how negative their prognosis, rather than the passive, helpless ones. For hope gives us energy, it gives us our fighting spirit. Hope also implies that wherever there is life, there is the possibility of change. The cells in our bodies are constantly dying, but within that death there can be great hope, as our cells are also being constantly reborn. So the opportunity for transformation is ever-present. If we deeply believe that we will heal, then that message will be conveyed to our very cell structure.

However, the road to discovering hope and love is not an easy one. The very problems we are dealing with in ourselves are there because we have been unable to confront or acknowledge them on a conscious level. Having become repressed, the energy then tries to find a means of expression through the body, to show us we are not in a balanced state. So here we now are, attempting to get well, yet in the process having to unravel the contents of a well-buried unconscious! And yet at the same time, if the willingness is there, this can be a tremendous opportunity to 'spring-clean the house' and discover new meaning in life. Illness or disease of any kind indicates constricted or traumatised energy, whereas health implies a state of free and peaceful energy. If we participated, no matter how unknowingly, in getting ill, then we can also participate in getting well. Discovering how and why the energy first became traumatised means discovering a deeper layer of ourselves. As Sun Bear expresses in *Healers on Healing*:

> The most common blocks are the negative attitudes that a lot of people carry around all the time. These blocks must be overcome for healing to occur. . . . In order to become totally healed, a person has to throw out hatred, envy, jealousy, and other destructive attitudes and feelings. Although such factors start within the mind, they quickly manifest in the body, becoming a stiff shoulder, a sluggish liver, cancer, or other illnesses. I believe that all genuine healing addresses the problem of unblocking negativities in one way or another.

In order to overcome the blocks, the negative attitudes and patterns that we have created, we first have to acknowledge that they are there. In so doing we often discover a 'Pandora's Box' of related incidents, pains, fears, long-standing resentments, unexpressed grief, anger, deep insecurities and confusion, as well as parts of our development that were left behind at the times of those incidents. Issues such as shame ('You ought to be ashamed of yourself', said a few too many times in childhood), abandonment or betrayal (as can occur in children at times of divorce or parental death), or repression ('Never mind dear,' when you really did mind and needed to express your feelings, but to do so simply created misunderstanding or violence). All these stay with us, influencing our actions and behaviour, our attitudes and our responses, and slowly affecting us on a physical level.

In learning to love ourselves we need to accept and even embrace all those aspects of ourselves that are shadowy, frightening and powerful. Remember how scared we used to be as children to go into a dark room, for we were sure we saw a monster lurking in the corner? And then when the light was put on we realised it was just our old teddy bear sitting in a chair? It's the same with those threatening monsters in our unconscious. We think they are much worse than they really are because they are hidden in the dark, but when we shine the light on them we find they are not so bad, not so hard to deal with, that we can actually love and forgive them quite easily. It is not always necessary to go back to our childhood for us to see the beginning of our patterns, for even if they did start there we may not remember them. We actually need only look back through the previous few months, at the most a year or two, to see examples of our behaviour that are repressed, angry, judgmental or fearful. And if we take any one of these attitudes and probe further, seeking the source, then we will find our way back to the more hidden issues.

Does it really make a difference which of the various techniques of healing or therapy we choose to follow? Is it not the faith in the technique, the faith in the practitioner, and the faith in ourselves that makes the difference? Should we not just find the technique that we feel most compatible with, and are thus able to have faith in? We will always be hearing miraculous stories about this or that cure, for there are innumerable methods available. Yet each one of them seems to be effective only with some people and not with all. One cancer patient told me that if she followed what everybody was telling her then she would be reduced to eating one carrot a day – and even carrots were frowned on by some! It is important to learn how to discriminate, for there will be many people wanting to help and do things for us, or offering 'fool proof' methods of healing. Some of these techniques will help by alleviating pain or tension, or by enabling us to go deeper inside ourselves, but no one thing can do it all. It is our bodies that will be doing the healing, not the therapy. And if we really listen to all the stories of cures that we are told, then what we are actually hearing is that the body can make use of any technique or method that we choose, as long as we believe in it.

No one else can smile for us, no one can breathe for us, and in the same way no one else can heal us. Healing is a faculty that we have within ourselves for our own use, it is not something that can be given to us from the outside. It is the power of the cells to regenerate when we are cut, of the immune system to destroy invading antigens, of the heart to mend after experiencing deep grief. The reality is that surgery, drugs, massage, acupuncture, herbs, crystals and so on, do not heal, but they do help create the environment in which we are able to contact our own healing energy. The various techniques assist in removing the barriers that are stopping us from being able to heal ourselves and they can stimulate our own desire to heal, but they are not the healing itself. That comes from within. In *The Healer's Hand Book* it says,

> There are many paths up a mountain. They will all get us there, but no one path is the only way to go. Each of us has to find our own way. There are signposts that can point us in the right direction but it is we who have to climb the rocks, cut down the jungle, or traverse the chasms. Exploring the various maps as we go is a way of getting to know our terrain. We can be warned of some of the pitfalls that lie ahead, aided when we fall into difficulties, and gently steered back on course when we lose direction. Understanding our mountain and what it is made of, reading the guidelines those who have gone before us have left, and learning to identify the signs along the way, all help our journey to be a smoother one.

A good therapist is someone who knows that he or she is not doing the healing, but that it is the energy inside each one of us that will move towards wellness or not, depending upon our motivation. So if we find we are searching for answers or cures in other people or in techniques, then we should consider if we are going in the right direction. To quote *The Healer's Hand Book* again:

> No one else can do this for us, we are the only ones who can deal with our selfish desires, our confusion or our hopelessness. There is a tendency to believe that some great external experience will some-how change us, will transform our consciousness and we may spend years chasing after this ultimate experience. But the mountain that has to be climbed is inside us.

A technique is like the words on a page. The words are not the meaning itself, just as a technique is not the healing. We have to find what is right for us, and trust in that. In our path towards wholeness one of the guidelines we can follow is what Dr Suzanne Kabasa has called the 'Three Cs'. They are challenge, commitment and control. With the first one we are able to approach our difficulties and stresses as challenges and opportunities, rather than being overcome by them. This is the development of hope versus hopelessness and passivity. With challenge comes commitment, the faith to see something through no matter how hard it gets, the sense of having meaning and purpose to our lives. This is the intent and willingness to go forward, combined with true vision. Having control means not being the victim of illnesses or problems, but feeling in control of the situation, able to make choices and decisions, and in this way to take responsibility for our own state of wellness.

The feeling that we can have control, that we are not just a victim of circumstances, is vital for the healing relationship to work. It is our bodies that are sick, and it is up to us to find the way to our own healing. Our own way of doing things may be different from someone else's. It may mean carrying on as normal and letting God heal us, it may mean relaxing or meditating, it may mean following a special diet, or it may mean taking a handful of pills every day. It is what it feels like to us that is important, not what it feels like to our doctors or well-meaning friends, who naturally want us to follow the path they feel is best for us. If we don't trust our doctors or therapists, or trust the treatment they are prescribing, then we need to have the courage to say so. It greatly helps if we feel that the person who is treating us also loves us and can therefore respect and work with our wishes.

In Chapter 1 we saw how what we are now is a result of all that has happened to us in the past, and our reactions and responses to that. This is the law of cause and effect, or karma. But karma is not a fixed state: it is constantly moving and shifting, depending on how we are dealing with ourselves and our actions. We have free choice at all times to change our attitudes, to no longer react to situations in the same ingrained way but to find new and more constructive responses. Then the results of our actions are free to change, to move. For instance, if we tend to be habitually nagging or complaining, then we will constantly see our world as a place full of flaws, out to attack us or to make our lives a misery. We will be miserable as a result, people will not enjoy being with us, and our bodies may become arthritic, stiff or even ulcerous. However, if we have the courage to see why we are so negative and what the underlying insecurities or fears are, and to begin to deal with these constructively, then we might find we start appreciating simple things like a bird singing, or the kind gesture of a girl at the supermarket checkout. Slowly our lives can become more loving, and our physical pains might also begin to recede. The choice is ours. The future grows out of our present thoughts and attitudes, and we have the power to change those thoughts, however deeply ingrained they may be, at any time.

Our understanding of life, our approach to it and our attitude towards ourselves and others, determines, to a very large extent, our state of ease or disease.

That does not mean that we should be blaming ourselves, or feeling intense guilt for not being aware of our hidden attitudes. This is very important, for it is easy to become overwrought with thinking we are to blame, yet obviously we do not consciously want to be ill. The patterns are on the unconscious level, they have been accumulating over a long period of time and are the result of our life experiences. Accepting this means that instead of guilt we see a challenge, an opportunity for change. By recognising what it is that we have been perpetuating, we can now focus on what is needed in order to move forward. Developing awareness and then creating a more positive attitude, one that is loving and compassionate towards ourselves, is the first step. Next we need to pay attention to what is happening in every minute of the day, so that we are not repressing or denying our feelings any more. This takes a deep commitment and intention, the willingness to heal, and the willingness to deal with whatever that healing may involve.

Cancer has been called the greatest of gifts, that which can change our lives and enable us to find our full potential. Bernie Siegal calls pain and suffering 'God's reset button', as sickness is sometimes the only thing that will make us wake up to who we are and stimulate deep change. Until that time there is no real motivation to look within. But decay is necessary for new growth; disintegration is necessary for integration to take place. Illness makes us ask what's it all about, why are we here, what is the purpose of life if we just fall ill and die? We spend all our time making money or raising children, when we cannot even take any of it with us when we leave! And we have spent little or no time finding out who we are, making friends with ourselves, or making friends with our world. We have no idea what goes on just below the surface in our own being.

Developing a healing relationship implies taking time to develop a relationship with ourselves, one in which we are honest, open, forgiving, accepting, loving and releasing. It may mean that we learn inner conscious relaxation, that we pray or meditate; maybe we go through psychotherapy or counselling; or we change our eating habits so that we become aware of what we are taking into our bodies. It might be that we join a support group. We may drop old friends and make new ones, or change the basis of old relationships so that they serve us better. In this way we are re-evaluating our attitudes and patterns. All or some of these actions can result as we shift our approach from looking outwards for answers to looking inwards.

Healing in this way also means coming to terms with our own death, with our own impermanence. It is the acceptance that all things are impermanent, that there is nothing we can hold on to that will stay the same, nothing that we can rely on except ourselves. And we will only be here as long as we are here. This acceptance can be a very positive and life-changing event, for it puts things in their proper perspective, helping us sort out our priorities. Does it really matter if we have lost our hair through chemotherapy treatments? Is it not more important that we are able to share our love with others? Is not the quality of our lives, the depth, meaning and love that can fill them, more important than how long or short our lives may be? Is not making peace with ourselves, our loved ones, and our death more important than worrying about what other people might be thinking about us? Only when we have made such peace can healing really occur, and only then can we even begin to help someone else find their peace. So rather than thinking that we are dying, and thus giving up, we can acknowledge that of course we are going to die, as everyone will, but in the process we are very much alive.

At the same time as saying this, it is important to understand that we all change and move at our own pace and in our own time. It is not something that can be forced, and we may not be ready yet to deal with such topics. The fear of change is enormous: it is the fear of letting go of the familiar in exchange for the unknown. We have to be very patient with ourselves. If we are confronting a serious illness then it may be quite a while before we are ready to look at personal issues. If we are dealing with smaller and simpler difficulties, the motivation might not be enough to make us look very far inside, only enough to solve our immediate situation. When we are ready, and when the motivation is strong enough, then the way through will appear. We will go forward and we will fall back, over and over again. And we will need more patience, and more love, and more acceptance. Slowly the body will heed our efforts and reflect our growing strength, determination and courage. It will move with our freer self-expression and respond to our inner probings. But it takes time.

As we make the journey to freedom from our traumatised state, we can be likened to a chicken trying to emerge from its shell. For that young chick the shell around it must feel like cast iron, like a suit of armour that it has to prise its way out of. It is natural for us to want to help by peeling away the shell and thus allowing the chick to be free. But if we do, the chick will die. It needs the strength it gains from breaking free of the shell in order to live, and it needs to do it by itself. We are like that chick. Our anger, guilt, fear, insecurity, shame and all our hidden monsters make up our shells, holding us back from experiencing true freedom. Breaking free is not easy, and no one else can do it for us. But if we have the courage to do it, then the strength and understanding we gain is the true healing.

'Healing is a total, organismic, synergistic response that must emerge from within the individual if recovery and growth are to be accomplished. Healing is creative, bringing forth patterns and connections that did not exist before,' says Emmet Miller in *Healers on Healing*. In other words, healing touches all the aspects of our lives, going far beyond being just the cure of a malady. It is a recognition that the illness itself is simply a way for the body to deal with underlying imbalanced or traumatised energies. Healing is the resolution of those imbalances. It is a discovery of our real purpose. We often hear stories of extraordinary remissions that take place, yet if we look closely it should not be so extraordinary. A remission is a re-mission, a re-discovery of our mission or purpose, and the healing that discovery gives us is greater than any illness we may have. Healing on this level does not necessarily mean we are suddenly able to get out of a wheelchair and walk again. It means we are healed within ourselves and can accept that, if being in the wheelchair is where we are meant to be, then that is fine.

In *Healing into Life and Death*, Stephen Levine says,

Healing, like grace can be somewhat disorientating in its early stages. It is a breaking through of the old to reveal the ever new. Healing, like grace, always takes us toward our true nature. Indeed, healing is not somewhere we are going, but a discovery of where we already are – a participation in the process unfolding moment to moment. Many of us pray for a miracle when all else has failed. We wish for grace to descend upon us. But grace comes from within. Grace arises when the work of healing is in process.

So healing does not necessarily produce a long and healthy life, or even the release of some symptoms, or any of the normal guidelines we think of as implying a cure. What it does do is bring together our intention with our thoughts, our feelings, our spirit and our bodies, so that an integrated understanding of what we need to do emerges. In this way we become free of the limitations that are holding us back, free of the repressions, and we can live more complete and aware lives. Ultimately there are no limitations, other than the ones we ourselves impose.

CHAPTER 8

The Way Through

Our distance from Heaven is in proportion to the measure of our self-love. EMANUEL SWEDENBORG

WHEN exploring our patterns of behaviour and the recurring events in our lives we soon see that nothing is actually accidental; even though on the surface there appears to be no meaning, when we dig a bit deeper we find there is an underlying theme, a timing and a purpose to all the various situations that we encounter. As we saw in Chapter 2, nature is never haphazard; there is an ongoing order and purpose present at all times throughout the natural world. It is when we become separated from nature, when we become so wrapped up in the world of materialism and achievement, that we forget we are actually an integral part of the flow of life. In this way we lose touch with both nature and with the natural rhythm and purpose in ourselves.

If we reconnect with that rhythm then we see how all things have their place, that all things happen exactly as they are meant to. Even if we do not fully understand why things happen, or why things happen in the way that they do, we can still tune into an understanding that goes beyond the immediate situation to the bigger picture, the more objective picture of life as a whole. From this viewpoint we see that we attract to us everything that it is necessary for us to experience at this particular time, whether it be a broken bone, the end of a relationship, an accident or the loss of a job. If we can rise above our subjective involvement and look down from above, as it were, to view the objective whole, then we see that what is happening to us is both a reflection of what we are manifesting for ourselves at this time, and something we need to experience in order for other things to manifest.

It would appear that we attract the negative in order to understand and integrate the positive, for one cannot come without the other; in every negative situation, whatever it may be, there is inherent in it a positive aspect. As we integrate the positive, so we no longer need the negative – its purpose is complete and it is free to go. If we were to write a list of all the qualities of the enlightened mind, of the mind that has reached the highest level of evolution in terms of consciousness, then we could put beside it a list of all the qualities of the unenlightened mind: the flip side. In this way we would be able to see that whatever negative or unenlightened event is happening to us also has a positive, enlightened aspect, and that this positive aspect is the real reason for us attracting the negative. If we are able to integrate the positive flip side inherent in the negative, then we can strike that negative aspect off the list as having been completed.

In realising that there is an underlying purpose to life, that all is not arbitrary but actually has direction, then we recognise that everything we are going through is there in order for us to realise this purpose further. Although as human beings we seem to have reached a level of physical evolution that is highly refined and versatile, one that does not necessarily need to improve too much, it appears that we still have a very long way to go in the evolution of consciousness. It may sometimes be hard to imagine, but each one of us is capable of profound and radical change within ourselves, change that can lead us to the higher states of wisdom, compassion, insight and unconditional love.

This is due to the intelligence which is present in every single cell of our being. We are all an integral part of the creative and natural world. There is a knowingness, connected to the intelligence of pure consciousness. Through our intelligence we have the power to change, to go beyond that which we think we are, to that which we have never experienced before. All around us we can see nature fulfilling itself, from the tiny acorn becoming a giant oak tree, to a small weed finding its way to the light through six inches of concrete. Life is constantly aiming at its own fruition. We are the only ones who hold ourselves back from fulfilment, for the very essence of our being is actually already free.

When we begin on the healing path, and especially when we use such methods as relaxation and meditation, we are opening ourselves to our inner intelligence, creating the space for our blocks and patterns to be released. For is it not our highest purpose to go beyond that which we think we are? To evolve in consciousness to higher states of enlightenment? To rediscover a sense of oneness with the infinite? In remembering our movement from the infinite to the finite at conception, is it not our purpose to rediscover the infinite within the finite, and finally to see that there is no difference between the two?

If this is the case, then we can presume that everything that happens to us is a part of that journey, one of discovering the divine within ourselves, no matter how hard it may be. For instance, depression and hopelessness are very common diseases, rooted in a sense of our having no purpose beyond birth and death. This feeling of purposelessness can be exceedingly destructive, even leading to suicide. Yet it can also be what inspires us to go on further. As Reshad Feild puts it in *Here to Heal*,

> The road that leads to the Truth is steep and, at times, precipitous. Indeed it does require tremendous patience and perseverance to keep on going when it seems that all the odds are against us, when there is nothing left to hold on to except that inner cry, that burning question as to why we exist at all.

As the external is a reflection of the internal, and the internal is affected by the external, so the events in our lives are connected to our inner state of being and are the very means we can use. All the factors that come together at conception and are built into us during gestation, as well as all the hindrances and difficulties that we encounter in life, these are the stepping stones that can lead us across the river from ignorance to wisdom. Our choice is how we deal with them. We may get stuck on the first stone, may lose our balance and fall, may be overcome by the distance involved and not even make an attempt to start; or we may have the courage to continue crossing despite all odds. We do have a purpose for being here, but we also have the choice to respond to this purpose or not – we have free will. Each hindrance has a hidden beauty: the greater understanding and freedom we can realise. By finding that beauty, we discover that there never was a hindrance. To quote once more from *Here to Heal*,

> True healing means the healing of the illusion that we are separate from the One Reality – a realisation that has slipped from our grasp. Healing means 'to become whole', to be one with our Creator as we

were at the beginning. It is what is meant by the words in the Bible, 'to be healed of our sins', for a sin is really only a *lack*, a lack of knowledge, a state of sleep and forgetfulness. What a pity if we were to pass through this life in such a state!

This state of sleep and forgetfulness is due to the ignorance of separation, the belief that we are all independent of each other. Normally our energy is consumed in the preservation of our ego, in supporting, maintaining and protecting our separate existence. We react to chaos and pain as if they came from outside of us, are being imposed upon us. We feel threatened by situations, and constantly blame others for everything we are experiencing. Our only means of coping with this world view is by escaping, ignoring or fighting back. Fear arises when this existence is threatened in any way.

When we can let go of the fear, even if only for a moment, then we can experience a tremendous freedom. For fear is false evidence appearing real, it is the delusion that this 'I' we spend so much time defending and protecting is an actual reality. Letting go of the fear enables us to see that there is a relationship between subject and object, between ourselves and other; that nothing exists independently, but all is inter-related; that it is our own mental projections being reflected back into our mind which are causing us so much suffering, not something from outside of us.

Pain and suffering are not the same thing. The existence of pain and pleasure is inherent to life; how it affects us is based on our reaction or response. Our suffering is a reaction to the pain, not the pain itself. A reaction is a re-acting, the repetition of behaviour that holds us in a limited mind set. To respond is to be creative, to act with an open mind, to create new possibilities within every moment.

In integrating this understanding we enter a state of ease and freedom, for our ego-centred and self-preserving needs become less dominant. When we release fear then we can give and love without losing anything. Through such love we find freedom from pain and suffering. Unconditional love is love without limitations, boundaries or conditions. The love is constant, it is not dependent on specific needs being fulfilled.

When there is no fear we are free to love in this way. In penetrating the nature of unconditional love we find that we can no longer make judgments and define limitations; therefore everything is exactly as it is meant to be. A caterpillar looks beautiful with all its textures and colours and shapes and hairs and legs. It is an exquisite caterpillar, perfect as it is. Can we therefore say it is more perfect when it becomes a butterfly? When it reaches a higher level of evolution? If it is not possible to measure perfection, then neither can we measure imperfection. We cannot say that one person is more sick than another. If we do, that is simply a reflection of our relative understanding. What is happening is as it is, not to be fought and resisted, but to be accepted and loved. Unconditional love does not distinguish between one experience of suffering and another, or between one expression of happiness and another.

In order to let go of the fear there needs to be this recognition and integration of the various aspects of our being. Just as a lotus flower grows out of the mud, so too the awakened mind grows out of that which is unawakened. The mud in ourselves is all the repressed and unacknowledged monsters in our unconscious, all the pain, anger, frustration, guilt, shame and abandonment issues that we carry around with us. The lotus flower not only grows out of this but it actually cannot grow without the mud, it has its roots firmly planted in it. In other words, we need our negative qualities in order to grow and become free; they are the very means through which we can develop. Accepting and loving our mud enables us to begin to grow our flower. And let us not deceive ourselves, for the mud is sticky, thick, lumpy, heavy and not easy to wash off or to find our way through!

The limitations we impose upon ourselves are therefore the ones of thinking we cannot get through this mud, all that it is far too overwhelming and impossible to find a way of coping with it all. We may try to ignore the mud and to focus only on the flower, in which case the flower will lack colour and brilliance – it will fade and die quickly. It needs the nourishment of the mud below to be a strong flower. If we accept that the mud is real, not to be ignored but to be welcomed with open arms, we can start removing our limitations. Then the desire to become free of the limitations becomes a priority, not just so that physical health may be maintained but so that psychological and emotional health can also be experienced.

Our limitations or blockages manifest themselves as dis-satisfaction or unhappiness, pain and disease (dis-ease). By recognising the process that goes from thought or feeling into form we can learn how to release the energy before it becomes physical, before it appears as illness or disease. As we respond to our inner patterns and take full responsibility for them, we can discover a new level of healing within. To be responsible means the ability to respond, so as we learn to respond to ourselves then our inner purpose can begin to make itself known.

To help us get in touch with our healer within, we need to be quiet, to find the space inside where we are at peace. We do this in order to evaluate what is happening in our lives: to see if there are issues we are negating or repressing, or if there are issues we have not acknowledged that are beginning to affect us physically. When we become ill we have more time to go within to communicate with ourselves and to see what it is that is happening, what it is that we need to do in order to become well. Through means such as inner conscious relaxation, guided visualisation and meditation we can gather all the various parts of ourselves together and find wholeness. *The Healer's Hand Book* says,

> Most of us think of relaxing as stretching out in an armchair, putting our feet up and letting the world go by without our interference for at least a few minutes. Our body might thus be eased, but to allow our mind to also relax is not so simple. There is normally a constant chatter going on, filling every space available, and it is not possible to try and stop this, for that very trying is still the mind at play. Instead we have to redirect our energy away from the mind and let go of the trying. As we relax we lose ourselves as we normally are and find ourselves in a new way.

Deep relaxation is now being used in many hospitals and healing centres to strengthen the immune system, to lower blood pressure, to release the tension in the muscles and to enable a deeper level of self-awareness to develop. The heartbeat slows down as we experience inner peace, as does the production of stress hormones. At the same time there is increased mental clarity and awareness and an easing of emotional tensions, anxieties, irritation and depression. Due to being quiet and peaceful within ourselves, insecurity and self-doubts begin to recede. We saw in Chapter 1 how stress can lower our resistance to disease, as can the accumulation of negative thinking patterns and attitudes. Now we see how during relaxation and medi-tation our resistance to disease is increased. It has been shown in many studies that yogis or those who practise meditation regularly can reduce their incidence of cardiovascular and nervous diseases by up to 80 per cent.

When we are truly relaxed healing can occur naturally, for we release the fear that was holding us in a state of tension. Much of the contents of our Pandora's Box may come up while we are trying to practise meditation, but in this state we are able to simply acknowledge and release without becoming involved. This is due to the presence of dispassion, the ability to move outside circumstances and to see them clearly. In meditation we tune into this more creative and dispassionate process of perception. Responding from this quiet centre our attitude becomes balanced, free of ego, and able to be objective and non-judgmental. The act of quietening the mind is a tool we can use to find the stillness within where there is no suffering.

The development of dispassion also furthers the development of compassion, the understanding that we are all one, that there is no difference or separation between us. As Father Thomas Merton has said, 'Compassion is a keen awareness of the interdependence of all living things which are all involved in one another and are all a part of one another.' Compassion is the objective expression of unconditional love, where we are motivated through the depth of our empathy and under-standing. It is beyond thoughts of 'I' or 'me'. It enables complete forgiveness to take place of both ourselves and of others, as we realise that hurt only occurs out of the ignorance of separation or duality, and we can forgive ignorance.

The particular relaxation or meditation technique that we use is not important. Each technique varies only in the methods it employs to quieten the mind, whether it be watching the breath, visualisation, or the repetition of a mantra (sound). The method is simply a prop that the mind can take hold of and direct its energy towards. In this way, we are able to focus and quieten the mind as it becomes free of distraction. It is not the object that is important, so much as the focusing. As this can take time to develop we should always have an attitude of lovingly accepting whatever we are capable of doing, not one of judging ourselves against others, or against where we would like to be.

Being quiet is not a natural state for most Westerners, and we will find considerable resistance within ourselves as we try to practise. For instance, it is not always easy for us to sit in a meditation posture on the floor, but rather than using this as an excuse not to meditate let us find an appropriate chair to sit on, or even lie down. Making friends with our relaxation or meditation practice is essential so that we do not see it as an enemy, but rather as a companion on the path to healing and self-awareness. Meditation is not a removal from the world, but is an active participation in understanding the world more deeply, by understanding ourselves more deeply. In the words of Thich Nhat Hanh:

Meditation is to be aware of what is going on – in our bodies, in our feelings, in our minds, and in the world. Each day 40,000 children die of hunger. The super-powers now have more than 50,000 nuclear warheads. Yet the sunrise is beautiful, and the rose that bloomed this morning is a miracle. Life is both dreadful and wonderful. To practice meditation is to be in touch with both aspects. Please don't think we have to be solemn in order to meditate. In fact, to meditate well, we have to smile a lot.

Included in this chapter are details of two practices. One is a guided visualisation that is designed to help us contact the inner causes and conflicts that are manifesting in our bodies. By entering into the body itself we can find out what it is trying to tell us and what we need to do so we may become healed and free. Then there is a meditation for developing loving kindness and compassion. In this practice we first have to develop love towards ourselves, and then we can expand it outwards to others. By using these two practices we can begin to find our own path to physical and emotional wholeness. These two practices are available on a cassette tape called 'Metta' by Debbie Shapiro, distributed by Element Books. For address, see p.200.

Inner Healing Visualisation

It is best to either read this practice on to a cassette tape so we can play it back to ourselves, or to have a friend read it and guide us through. It should be read slowly, allowing time between each instruction, taking approximately thirty minutes for the whole practice. It can be done alone or in a group. Before starting, have some paper and a pen close by.

To do this practice we should lie down with a thin pillow

under our head and a blanket covering us. Our arms are by our sides, hands upwards. Our feet are slightly apart. Our eyes are closed.

This is a guided visualisation to enable us to contact and communicate with our bodies from the inside. This is not always easy. If we are sick, are in pain or are experiencing some form of physical difficulty, we can use this practice to go within to find out what it is that this part of our being needs us to do, in order for there to be freedom. However, we may find our bodies shy or resistant to talking with us at first. Our bodies express the unconscious and unacknowledged patterns within us, and there may be suspicion of us now saying we want to bring these patterns into the conscious mind. If we persevere, we will find the communication opens and we will be able to understand ourselves, and what is happening to us, more deeply.

During the practice we allow any answers to our questions to arise spontaneously. The body may use the dream language of the unconscious to convey a message to us, so we accept whatever images arise even if we do not understand them at the time.

Now we take a deep breath and let it out through the mouth. Make it a deep sigh. And again. Letting it out through the mouth. And we begin to relax. We begin to sink into the floor, becoming heavy and peaceful.

Now we take our attention to the feet and begin to work upwards, from the feet through our legs, relaxing any tension that we find. Breathing into the tension and letting it go. Relaxing.

Up through the pelvis, the lower back, the middle back and the upper back. Breathing into the tension and letting go.

Up through the abdomen and the chest. Relaxing deeply. Letting go.

From the hands, up the arms, into the shoulders, and then the neck. Breathing and relaxing.

Then we relax all the facial muscles and the head. We take a deep breath and completely let go. We are fully relaxed and at peace.

Now we take a few minutes to follow our breathing as the breath comes in and out of our belly. We count at the end of each breath, starting at ten, then nine, then eight, and down to zero. Letting go. We repeat this counting of the breaths once more.

Now we imagine we are getting smaller and smaller, until we are so small we can come in and walk around inside our own bodies. We come inside and then find our way to an area that is in pain, is suffering in some way and needs healing, an area that is not happy. This may also be a psychological or emotional pain if we want.

When we get there we start to explore what we have found, the particular tissue structure of this area, and the environment.

What shape is this area? Is it round, or is it long and thin?

How big is this area? Is it so small we can walk around it, or is it so big that we cannot see the other side? Allow the images to come.

What does it feel like? What texture is it? Is it soft and spongy, or hard, or like rubber?

What colour is it? Is it red, or dark-coloured, or light and almost translucent?

What temperature is it? Is it so hot that we cannot touch it, or is it nice and cool?

How old is this area? Has it been like this for a long time, or is it quite recent?

We allow the images of this area and the surrounding tissue structure to emerge.

Most importantly, do we feel safe being here? Is it all right to be here, or would it feel safer to back off a little, to take a bit more time getting to know this area before we get any closer? We do whatever feels right. We can leave at any time, or go to another part of the body if that feels better. We trust our own instinct to know what to do.

If the communication is open, then we can continue asking questions to find out what it feels like from the inside. Whatever images come into the mind we explore them, follow them, allow them to communicate with us, to become real, even if we do not understand them. We watch what our reaction is, if we are being fearful, judgmental, and so on. As we explore further we begin to realise how much energy there is here and how we can communicate with that energy.

We can ask why this area of pain or tension is like this. What happened to make it this way? And when? We allow the answers to come without discrimination.

And then we can find out what is needed here. What can we now do to enable this part of ourselves to be free?

What action do we need to take? What do we need to work

with or change in our lives so we may be healed?

We may find that this area is ready to go and it just needed our acknowledgment and recognition first. Or we may find that there are certain things we need to do. Each time we do this practice the answers will be different, so we allow time for the area of pain to speak to us in its own way.

When we are ready to leave, we acknowledge what has happened by saying thank you, promising to act on whatever has been asked of us, and making arrangements to be back at another time. This is very important. For our bodies to trust us we have to show that we are being sincere and honest, as well as respectful of the body itself.

We slowly find our way out of our bodies and grow big enough to fit back into ourselves again. We take a deep breath. We may wish to write down everything that has happened. As with dreams, we may not understand it all, but we let the images or words become a part of our lives until the meaning becomes clear.

We can repeat this practice often to develop an open communication with what is happening inside, and to learn how we can be free of that which is holding us back.

The Metta Bhavana – Loving Kindness Meditation

This is a meditation practice that lasts approximately twenty-five to thirty minutes. It can be read on to a cassette tape so that we can play the tape to ourselves, or we can have a friend read the instructions to us. Approximately five to seven minutes should be allowed for each of the five stages of the meditation. It can be done alone or in a group setting.

To start with, we find a comfortable sitting position, whether on the floor or on a chair, with the spine upright, the hands on the thighs or in the lap, and the eyes closed. Take a deep breath and relax.

1. This is the first stage of the Metta Bhavana practice, the development of loving kindness and compassion. To truly practise unconditional love we have to start by loving ourselves just as we are, fully and unconditionally. This is not always easy, but we cannot truly love others until we have this love for ourselves. We have to look at all that which is stopping us from loving ourselves, and be able to accept, forgive and be at peace

with that.

In this first stage we take our attention to the area of our heart, and then repeat to ourselves, 'May I be well, may I be happy, may all things go well for me.' Really allowing the feeling to grow within. We acknowledge all the opposing thoughts that come to mind – reasons why we should not be happy or not be well; feelings of guilt and shame, of not being worthy, or our inability to receive. And we continue repeating, 'May I be well, may I be happy, may all things go well for me' for the next few minutes. Letting the feeling in our hearts grow.

Allowing any feelings to emerge, we focus on loving ourselves. Let the love shine, let the forgiveness be there. 'May I be well, may I be happy, may all things go well for me.'

2. Now, in the second stage, we take our loving kindness and compassion and direct it towards a near and dear friend. We choose someone within twenty years of our own age and someone of the same sex, simply to avoid parental or romantic feelings, and to allow true unconditional love to develop. Holding this person in our hearts, and feeling the love we were feeling for ourselves now go towards this person, we repeat, 'May they be well, may they be happy, may all things go well for them.'

We feel the joy in our hearts and feel the love radiate throughout our being. 'May they be well, may they be happy, may all things go well for them.'

3. Now, in the third stage, we direct our loving kindness and compassion towards a neutral person, someone for whom we have neither positive nor negative feelings. We may not even know their name. We focus on this person and hold them in our hearts and let the unconditional love flow towards them. 'May they be well, may they be happy, may all things go well for them.'

Holding this neutral person in our hearts, we feel the love for the unknown, for in reality we are all one. 'May they be well, may they be happy, may all things go well for them.'

4. Now, in the fourth stage, we direct our loving kindness and compassion towards what is traditionally known as the enemy. An enemy is someone with whom we are experiencing negative communication. This may be a relative, friend, colleague or anyone else in our lives with whom all is not well, whether they are feeling it towards us or we towards them. We hold this person in our hearts and let our acceptance and love flow towards them. 'May they be well, may they be happy, may

all things go well for them.'

Remembering that pain is born out of ignorance and we can forgive ignorance, so we feel the love and compassion for this person. 'May they be well, may they be happy, may all things go well for them.'

5.   Now, in the fifth stage, we start by lining up these four people: ourselves, our friend, the neutral person and the enemy, and we feel such unconditional love towards all four that, if we were asked to pick one in preference over the others, we would not be able to do so. Our love is truly unconditional. Our loving kindness radiates equally to all four.

From these four we now begin to expand our loving kindness and compassion towards all beings. Slowly it radiates outwards from ourselves towards all those in our vicinity. Then outwards further, reaching out to all beings, so that we are unconditionally loving all, whether they be a murderer or a saint, realising there is no difference between ourselves and all other beings. We repeat, 'May all beings everywhere be happy, may all beings be well, may all things go well.'

We expand our loving kindness to all beings everywhere, in all directions of space. And we repeat, 'May all beings be at peace, and may I be at peace with all beings.'

Cassette Tape

These two practices, *Inner Healing Visualisation* and *Metta,* are available on cassette tape, along with other meditation and relaxation tapes, from the author. For information e-mail samadhi@compuserve.com.

Bibliography

Connelly, Dr Dianne M., *Traditional Acupuncture: the Law of the Five Elements*. Centre for Traditional Acupuncture Inc., Maryland.

Damian, Jonathan, *Wholistic Phenomenology*.

Dytchwald, Ken, *Bodymind*. Wildwood House.

Feild, Reshad, *Here to Heal*. Element Books.

Ferguson, Marilyn, *The Aquarian Conspiracy*. Jeremy Tarcher.

Harvey, John, *The Quiet Mind*. The Himalayan International Institute of Yoga Science and Philosophy, Honesdale, Pennsylvania.

King, Serge, *Imagineering for Health*. Quest Books.

König, Karl, *'Meditation on the Endocrine System'*.

LeShan, Lawrence, *How You Can Fight for Your Life*. M. Evans & Co. Inc., New York.

Levine, Stephen, *Healing into Life and Death*. Doubleday.

Regan, Georgina, and Shapiro, Debbie, *The Healer's Hand Book*. Element Books.

St John, Robert, *Metamorphosis*.

St Pierre, Gaston, and Shapiro, Debbie, *The Metamorphic Technique*. Element Books.

Siegel, Dr Bernie, *Love, Medicine and Miracles*. Harper and Row.

Yogananda, Paramahansa, *Collected Sayings*.

Index